CLINICAL TRIALS AND TRIBULATIONS

CLINICAL TRIALS AND TRIBULATIONS

GAYATHRI DE LANEROLLE

PETER PHIRI

ATHAR HAROON

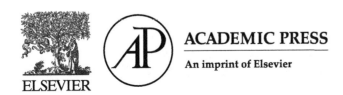

ACADEMIC PRESS

An imprint of Elsevier

ELSEVIER

Academic Press is an imprint of Elsevier
125 London Wall, London EC2Y 5AS, United Kingdom
525 B Street, Suite 1650, San Diego, CA 92101, United States
50 Hampshire Street, 5th Floor, Cambridge, MA 02139, United States
The Boulevard, Langford Lane, Kidlington, Oxford OX5 1GB, United Kingdom

Notices
Knowledge and best practice in this field are constantly changing. As new research and experience broaden our
understanding, changes in research methods, professional practices, or medical treatment may become
necessary.

Practitioners and researchers must always rely on their own experience and knowledge in evaluating and using
any information, methods, compounds, or experiments described herein. In using such information or methods
they should be mindful of their own safety and the safety of others, including parties for whom they have a
professional responsibility.

To the fullest extent of the law, neither the Publisher nor the authors, contributors, or editors, assume any liability
for any injury and/or damage to persons or property as a matter of products liability, negligence or otherwise, or
from any use or operation of any methods, products, instructions, or ideas contained in the material herein.

ISBN 978-0-12-821787-0

For information on all Academic Press publications
visit our website at https://www.elsevier.com/books-and-journals

Publisher: Stacy Masucci
Acquisitions Editor: G. Andre Wolff
Editorial Project Manager: R. Andrea Dulberger
Production Project Manager: Omer Mukthar Moosa
Cover Designer: Mark Rogers

Typeset by STRAIVE, India

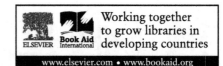

Contents

Chapter 11 Research governance and compliance management 215

Gayathri De Lanerolle, Peter Phiri, Athar Haroon, Heitor Cavalini,
and Kathryn Elliot

Chapter 12 Audits and inspections 219

Gayathri De Lanerolle, Peter Phiri, Athar Haroon, and Heitor Cavalini

Chapter 13 Patients and public support 233

Gayathri De Lanerolle, Peter Phiri, Athar Haroon, and Heitor Cavalini

Note from the authors:

We would like to acknowledge Ms Sana Sajid for helping us complete the administrative aspects of completing this book

The clinical research landscapes

Key messages
- Clinical trials have significantly evolved over the last century, with rapid advancements specifically in both the electronic and/or virtual delivery over the last 2 years
- Clinical trials have improved the evidence generation methods to better clinical practices over the last 50 years
- Epidemiology studies are an important aspect of the research landscape that could inform clinical trials and vice versa
- The historical challenges have been taken up by the researcher community as a 'lesson-learnt' to better manage and regulate clinical research
- Considerable overregulation of some areas needs to be taken into consideration when processes, regulations, and legislations are put in place

'The charm of history and its enigmatic lesson consist in the fact that, from age to age, nothing changes and yet everything is completely different.'

Aldous Huxley

1.1 A brief history

Clinical research is the foundation of medicine and is the most vital method used to improve healthcare by way of improving disease diagnosis, treatment, and management strategies. The clinical research landscape has had a fascinating journey over centuries, from the very first recorded clinical trial [1] of the modern era in 1747 by Dr. James Lind that successfully treated Scurvy amongst sailors. Lind systematically reviewed existing knowledge and provided a *real-time* treatment. Throught the evidence synthesis, Lind narrowed his treatment and compared the outcomes

Clinical Trials and Tribulations. https://doi.org/10.1016/B978-0-12-821787-0.00010-6

in 12 sailors. Whilst the British Navy did not employ the use of citrus fruit as a treatment for many decades due to the costs associated with tropical fruits at the time, the scientific community and patients appreciated the findings. The balance between economic evaluation, patient benefit, and policy implementation has only become more complicated in the present day, which persistently hinders healthcare outcomes.

Ethical considerations are key in human research and this became a prominent feature following the criminal medical experiments conducted by the Nazis during World War II. This resulted in the development of 10 fundamental principles to adhere to when conducting research on humans under the Nuremberg Code of 1949 and its extension, the Declaration of Helsinki of 1949, which was adopted in 1964 by the World Medical Association. Clinical equipoise featuring the balance between ethical and scientific principles became an important aspect to consider in order to assess the efficacy of novel interventions. The precepts of ethical guidelines from the Hippocratic Oath have widened the use of these principles practically by all those involved amongst clinical research professionals. The changes in clinical research itself have influenced the clinical profession where complexities around study delivery, coupled with the significant rise in population versus disease diagnosis, treatment, and/or long-term management, have led to the development of new professional roles. Thus, the research workforce is a multidisciplinary perpetuating profession that embodies research philosophies of ontology and epistemology to generate new knowledge and improve clinical practices. Hardy [2] theorised that ontology instructs epistemology issues that could assist with understanding both *knowledge* and *practice*.

Clinical trials have a turbulent history, although the scientific curiosity appears to be driven even further despite the complications. The Book of Daniel was the first document to show a clinical research experiment and dates back to 600 BC. The Babylonian King, Nebuchadnezzar, wanted to understand the health effects between a red meat and a vegetarian diet coupled with and without wine, respectively, over a period of 10 days. The strength of this study was the contemporaneous control group whilst the weakness was ascertainment and selection bias. Centuries later in 1537, Dr. Amborise Pare conducted another research study associated with use of egg yolk, rose oil, and turpentine to treat combat casualty wounds. Pare's observations noted there was better pain management with this mixture in comparison to the commonly used boiling oil method. The wounds reduced inflammation in comparison to those that were treated with burning oil. Pare's innovative wound care regime led to further experimentations over the 16th and 17th centuries which was often referred to as experimental medicine. Claude Bernard, in 1865, published a book called 'Introduction to the Study of Experimental Medicine' that emphasised the need to rethink their codes of practice and to use scientific methods. Bernard was the first to propose evidence-based standard of care and stipulated:

> *To learn we must necessarily reason about what we have observed, compare the facts, and judge them by other facts as controls.*

Bernard's publication made a case for the use of rigorous scientific methods to improve and validate clinical treatments. The idea of use of comparator groups in the form of a controlled to modern-day placebo effects as a core component of clinical trials. The world's first 'placebo' effect was assessed by Austin Flint in 1863 using rheumatic fever patients. Flint's study demonstrated symptoms of rheumatic fever that subsided over time which marked a shift in clinical practice where active treatment was more centralised.

A few decades later, the establishment of medical research institutions to lead and manage clinical research became prominent, alongside that of academic organisations and healthcare organisations. A key establishment during this period was the Medical Research Council (MRC) that conducted the world's first double-blind comparative clinical trial that evaluated Paulin, an extract of Penicillium Patulinum, on the common cold. This study took place between 1943 and 1944 across multiple centres in the United Kingdom. An initial trial of Patulinum to cure common colds had been conducted prior by the Royal Navy although unclear results were made available. Whilst Patulinum demonstrated to be ineffective, the MRC demonstrated the importance of scalability and inclusion of various participants from different parts of the United Kingdom.

This was followed-up with the infamous Dr. Austin Bradford Hill and Dr. Philip Hart's trial in 1946 to assess the use of Streptomycin on Tuberculosis. Dr. Marc Daniels was the trial coordinator and was responsible for registering the patients in the national coordinating centres. Each participating centre had allocated references, and if a patient was eligible to take part in the study, a hospital ED was arranged within the locality by Mrs Charlene Agnews, the very first clinical trial manager on record. Envelopes with allotted number series were used to randomise to either the control or streptomycin arm. The order of the envelopes was further randomised using random numbers. This team coordinated, designed, analysed, and reported the results of the study in The Lancet. The organisation of this trial was facilitated through the parliament act of tuberculosis agreed in 1911, which had used a model of outpatient clinics. The ethical review of the study was completed by the chairman of the oversight committee; Sir Geoffrey Marshall and the consultant physicians of the Royal Brompton Hospital were the first to start the patient screening procedures. This clinical trial is a landmark as it was noted as the first randomised controlled clinical trial that opened the door to a new era in clinical research, and in turn, in medicine.

Despite these positive strides, clinical trials did have a fall from grace amidst the use of Thalidomide by pregnant women. Thalidomide was developed by CIBA, a Swiss pharmaceutical company in 1953, and distributed by Chemi Grunenthal, a German pharmaceutical company, from 1956 onwards. Thalidomide was approved as a nonbarbiturate hypnotic sedative and was initially prescribed for many people with insomnia. During the 1950s, unlike the modern era where vigorous testing of drugs across multiple phases amongst human participants is a requirement, preclinical evaluation was sufficient for multipurpose use. As Thalidomide did not show any issues of dependency, this was prescribed as an antiemetic amongst women with morning sickness. The cost-effectiveness and wider availability of the Thalidomide allowed it to become a popular drug worldwide. However, in 1961, Dr. William McBride, an Obstetrician and Dr. Widukind Lenz, a Paediatrician and Geneticist, observed that Thalidomide use amongst pregnant woman was leading to congenital malformations such as amelia, phocomelia, syndactyly, underdeveloped long bones as well as cardiac abnormalities and aplasia of the appendix and gallbladder. These outcomes were mainly amongst women who took a single dose of Thalidomide between 34 and 49 days postmenstruation. Approximately 40% of the infants that were born from these women died within a year; this eventually led to Thalidomide being withdrawn from the market.

1.2   The 'clinical research' revolution

Clinical research was revolutionised simultaneously with discoveries and the growth in methodologies to test the novel interventions. As researchers developed new designs, clinical trials and nonclinical trials began to form a nomenclature based on a number of factors including the research question, objectives, and outcomes. Based on this, clinical research was primarily classified into observational and clinical trials, which could, in turn, be subcategorised further.

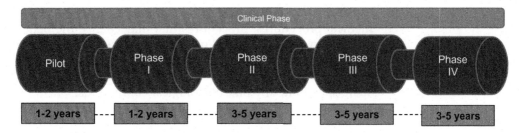

Fig. 1.1 The compositions within the clinical phase which take approximately 18–20 years, including the analyses period required prior to publication.

Clinical trials

Researchers gradually moved from traditional models of designing and evaluating novel interventions uniformly to systematically comparing and quantifying efficacy through a *phase I, II, III, and IV* (Fig. 1.1). This became a paradigm shift primarily for drug development using clinical trials. Clinical trials are categorised as experimental studies that could be controlled or uncontrolled. Controlled clinical trials comprise a control group that can be either randomised or nonrandomised. Nonrandomised trials often are designed as quasiexperimental, community, or field trials. Uncontrolled trials lack a control group and commonly report linear outcomes. During the development of medical devices, often clinical trials are either a registry or a phase II.

Conceptualisation of clinical trials

The conceptualisation of clinical trials refers to a group of complex tasks that together facilitate and clarify clinical outcomes considered vital to assess clinical effectiveness. The 'implementability' of trials, as they are conceived and conducted through their four phases, refers to the study design, execution, and reporting of clinical trials that may influence the ability to implement the evidence generated by that trial [3].

In summary, a clinical study involves research using human volunteers (also called participants in the clinical context and/or samples in the literature). Such studies aim, for instance, to increase medical knowledge, prove the effectiveness of specific drugs, materials, or techniques. There are two main types of clinical studies: clinical trials (also called intervention studies) and observational studies [4].

In a clinical trial, participants receive specific interventions according to a protocol and research plan designated by the researchers. These interventions can be medications, devices, medical procedures, procedures that may change the behaviour of participants and diets. Furthermore, clinical trials can make comparisons with existing drugs available for use with new drugs, or make comparisons of existing drugs with placebos, i.e., substances without any pharmacological compounds.

In the past 50 years, many clinical trials have been written and registered. However, more randomised and controlled studies [5] are needed. Such studies are considered to have the highest level of recommendation for clinical practice. Nevertheless, in the literature, there is still not enough data on how to effectively manage a clinical trial. Many clinical trials fail due to the lack of a structured, practical, and business approach to test management [6].

Good and efficient test management is a crucial factor amongst the key competences that are needed to provide high-quality tests. It is recognised that well-designed trials are the foundation for addressing important clinical questions; however, science alone is not enough to successfully deliver a trial. The main challenge is to establish and implement management systems and techniques that are effective and responsive to research needs [7]. Every clinical trial must be conducted exactly in the same way, regardless of size, scope, costs, or duration.

A metaanalysis that compiled the results from 114 multicentre studies [8] showed that 45% of the trials failed to reach 80% of the preestablished sample size. An important factor seen in the clinical trials that were successfully conducted was that they all hired a person with data management and research skills to compose the research group.

Furthermore, the Medical Research Custom, in another review, found that the cause of some trial failures may have been problems in the management and logistics of those trials, rather than scientific problems or issues with the design of the trials [9]. Francisco et al., in a broader analysis [8], questioned whether clinical trials should be planned and managed from the same perspective as a company, taking into account business management strategies. He also suggested that the execution of a successful trial should include 'marketing', 'sales', and 'continuous customer management'.

With this in mind, we can say that the good management of the study is not only linked to success in the scientific part but also in the logistics, feasibility, and costs of the research. This brings us to a crucial point where we can align good management in the pilot studies. When used properly, pilot and feasibility studies can provide sufficient methodological evidence about a study design, planning, and rationale. A good feasibility study [10] followed

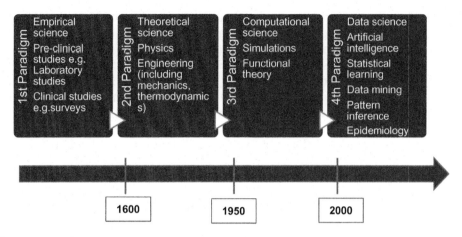

Fig. 1.2 Scientific paradigms.

by good management can avoid, or even eliminate, major errors such as increased uncalculated costs, sample loss, and time misspent by the medical team. Therefore, understanding and applying the most fit for purpose scientific paradigm is vital to accept or decline a hypothesis and then to conduct the process of answering the research question effectively (Fig. 1.2).

Epidemiology studies

Epidemiology studies have advanced over centuries and originally date back to the time of Hippocrates (460–377 BC). Hippocrates (Fig. 1.3) was determined to describe diseases by way of

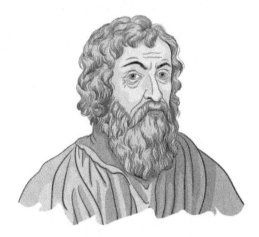

Fig. 1.3 Hippocrates.

incidence and mortality using a systematic method. The systematic approaches were further mentioned in Hippocrates's books *Epidemic I, Epidemic III* and *On Airs, Waters and Places* that describe disease incidence and prevalence. Hippocrates identified and defined *hot and cold disease*. Hot diseases were defined as any condition treated by cold treatments?, whilst cold diseases as those treated with hot treatments. Determining if a condition was hot or cold was a complex process and atomic theory was considered by Hippocrates. Hippocrates theorised of four atoms of earth, air, fire, and water. Using this theory, it was decided that diarrhoea was a hot disease requiring cold treatments such as fruits. Hippocrates also thought the human body comprised phlegm, yellow bile, blood, and black bile, based on earth and water atoms, fire and air atoms, fire and water atoms, and earth and air atoms, respectively. Illness was therefore hypothesised to have been caused by an imbalance of these components. Hippocrates contributed to the initial understanding of epidemiological concepts of observations and causal factors. Observations made in relation to disease occurrence, locality, and symptoms assisted with understanding the flue epidemics although the cause remained unknown until 1900, when Walter Reed showed mosquitos could be responsible.

Thomas Sydenham (1624–1689) furthered this work from an observational rather than a theoretical perspective. Sydenham studied at the University of Oxford medical school, and affiliated with the All Souls College where he became acquainted with Robert Boyle. Boyle sparked scientific curiosity within Sydenham, who approached diseases and epidemics using empirical approaches in the first instance. Sydenham wrote about disease observations without the use of traditional theories, which were published in 1676 within the book *Observations Medicae*. This book included classifications of plagues that incurred in London in 1660 and 1670 to describe three classes of fevers: continued fever, intermittent fever, and smallpox. Sydenham treated patients with smallpox with bed rest although Hippocrates theory was to use extensive bed covers and heat. Thus, it was no surprise when Sydenham's colleagues threatened to revoke his medical licence despite the positive public views and support. There were many young and open-minded physicians that agreed with Sydenham's empirical and unconventional approaches which led to the very first descriptions of psychological maladies. Sydenham also advanced many other lifestyle remedies such as the importance of a healthy diet, exercise, and airy spaces, which many other physicians did not support at the time.

In 1700s, James Lind used epidemiological theories of observation to understand scurvy amongst sailors. Whilst Lind's work was recorded as the first modern-day clinical trial, the treatment he tested was based on his observations of symptoms of scurvy patients such as bleeding gums and skin, putrid gums, weakness of the knees, muscular pain, and extreme weakness of the limbs that progressed over 4–6 weeks whilst at sea. Lind also observed that the symptoms worsened during poor weather and the dampness increased within the months of April, May, and June where there was an increase in rainy weather. Although the weather is not directly correlated to scurvy, Lind's theory does demonstrate that this could be the reason for some of the muscular pain. During Lind's time with the HMS Salisbury in 1747, the experiment was conducted with 12 sailors who appeared to have the same level of symptoms. The epidemiologic contribution Lind made was significant as the clinical observations and the use of an experimental design based on a specific population supported further work undertaken centuries later such as the work of John Snow, Louise Pasteur, Robert Koch, John Graunt, William Farr, Mary Mallon, Florence Nightingale, Edgar Sydenstricker, Edward Jenner, Ignaz Semmelweis, Benjamin Jesty, and Richard Doll.

1.3 Modern-day clinical research

The global clinical research landscape has changed significantly. The United States and the United Kingdom continue to be the clinical research giants influencing the global healthcare generation of new knowledge and practices with many other countries as China, Japan, India, and Germany increasing their footing steadily [11]. Equally, the use of the term 'clinical research' has equally evolved and no longer defines clinical trials alone.

Epidemiology studies and clinical trials have influenced modern-day medicine. Experimental designs have evolved significantly for both observational and interventional studies. With the influence of the COVID-19 global pandemic [12], clinical trials have further advanced in the manner in which they are designed, set up, managed, and delivered. The COVID-19 pandemic has been considered as a major global health threat reminding healthcare systems, policy-makers, and the general public the impact a rise in a disease could have in the absence of system preparedness and minimal availability of novel therapeutics that would aid reducing incidence, prognosis, and mortality [13]. The series of events that impacted a large proportion of countries had negative ramifications around delivering existing nonpandemic research. The pandemic highlighted the lack of suitable infrastructure to maintain research activities, as well the inadequate policies and regulations to rapidly setup and conduct clinical trials to gather data needed to improve prognosis, identification of treatments, and reducing mortality [14]. In addition, the pandemic provided an opportunity for increased awareness of clinical research and the importance of conducting efficient and effective clinical trials.

References

[1] Delanerolle G, Thayanandan T, Riga J, Griffiths J, Lawson J, Au-Yeung S, et al. Clinical trials: from problem child to the driving force of medical advancement. Br J Neurosci Nurs 2020;16(5). https://doi.org/10.12968/bjnn.2020.16.5.200.

[2] Hardy M. I know what I like and I like what I know': epistemology in practice and theory and practice again. Qual Soc Work 2016;15(5–6):762–78. https://doi.org/10.1177/1473325016654962.

[3] Cumpston MS, Webb SA, Middleton P, Sharplin G, Green S. Understanding implementability in clinical trials: a pragmatic review and concept map. Trials 2021;22:232. https://doi.org/10.1186/s13063-021-05185-w.

[4] Clinical Trials. Learn about clinical studies, https://clinicaltrials.gov/ct2/about-studies/learn.

[5] Yusuf S, Collins R, Peto R. Why do we need some large, simple randomized trials? Stat Med 1984;3(4):409–22. https://doi.org/10.1002/sim.4780030421.

[6] Farrell B, Kenyon S, Shakur H. Managing clinical trials. Trials 2010;11:78. https://doi.org/10.1186/1745-6215-11-78.

[7] Francis D, Roberts I, Elbourne DR, Shakur H, Knight RC, Garcia J, et al. Marketing and clinical trials: a case study. Trials 2007;8:37. https://doi.org/10.1186/2F1745-6215-8-37.

[8] Campbell MK, Snowdon C, Francis D, Elbourne D, McDonald AM, Knight R, et al. STEPS group: recruitment to randomised trials: strategies for trial enrolment and participation study. The STEPS study. Health Technol Assess 2007;11(48). https://doi.org/10.3310/hta11480. iii-ix-105.

[9] Medical Research Council. Clinical trials for tomorrow. London: MRC; 2003.

[10] Moher D, Glasziou P, Chalmers I, Nasser M, Bossuyt PMM, Korevaar DA, et al. Increasing value and reducing waste in biomedical research: who's listening? Lancet 2016;387(10027):1573–86. https://doi.org/10.1016/S0140-6736(15)00307-4.

[11] Catalá-López F, Alonso-Arroyo A, Hutton B, Aleixandre-Benavent R, Moher D. Global collaborative networks on meta-analyses of randomized trials published in high impact factor medical journals: a social network analysis. BMC Med 2014;12:15. https://doi.org/10.1186/1741-7015-12-15. 24476131. PMCID: PMC3913337.

[12] Rathod S, Pallikadavath S, Graves E, Rahman MM, Brooks A, Soomro MG, et al. Impact of lockdown relaxation and implementation of the face-covering policy on mental health: a United Kingdom COVID-19 study. World J Psychiatry 2021;11(12):1346–65. https://doi.org/10.5498/wjp.v11.i12.1346.

[13] Mayor N, Meza-Torres B, Okusi C, Delanerolle G, Chapman M, Wang W, et al. Developing a long COVID phenotype for postacute COVID-19 in a national

primary care sentinel cohort: observational retrospective database analysis. JMIR Public Health Surveill 2022;8(8), e36989. https://doi.org/10.2196/36989.

[14] Cavalini H, Qin Z, Zhen Y, Shi JQ, Shetty A, Neves V, et al. STOBE: a long-COVID syndromic study using real-world data in Brazil: Heitor Cavalini. Eur J Public Health 2022;32(3). https://doi.org/10.1093/eurpub/ckac131.189.

Further reading

Delanerolle G, Ebrahim R, Goodinson W, Elliot K, Shetty A, Phiri P. The emperors of scientific versatility that influenced clinical medicine; Dr Golding Bird and Nikola Tesla. Authorea; 2021 March 23. https://d197for5662m48.cloudfront.net/documents/publicationstatus/60024/preprint_pdf/28f8cc03167a10e4cb30150 d78b70474.pdf.

2

Clinical trials and epidemiology studies

Key messages

- Clinical trial design should include a clear outline of the hypothesis, research question, method for study delivery, and data collection
- Clinical trials and Epidemiology studies' evidence generation methods should have core documents of a statistical analysis plan (SAP), risk management document (RMD), and roles and responsibilities document (RRD)
- Regulations for Epidemiology studies and Clinical trials differ and as a result, the manner in which studies are set up and conducted will be specific
- Medical devices tested as part of clinical trials in the United Kingdom have specific regulations and legislations that should be followed by all external sponsors

2.1 Background

Clinical research is delivered at a hierarchical level as a clinical trial or an epidemiology study. Fundamentals of clinical trials [1] and epidemiology studies are similar although there are important differences in the manner in which these are conducted. Classification of the evidence generated could be ranked based on the strengths of their data quality. The starting point to these studies would be to start with robust clinical question with four essential components: Patient/Population or Problem, Intervention, Comparison, and Outcome (PICO). The PICO format is described below:

- Patient/Population or Problem: multiple considerations around the relevant cohort of patients and the primary clinical problem to resolve. This should include details such as age, gender, race or ethnicity, body mass index (BMI), geographical location, and health status.

- Intervention: the plan of diagnostic or treatment strategy including medication or surgical procedures.
- Comparison: a comparator intervention, either as a diagnostic test, medication, or surgical procedure, which would measure against a gold standard or a placebo. The comparative treatment may sometimes be a 'wait and watch' category which is often used in longitudinal studies.
- Outcomes: outcomes are the consequences of the exposures associated with the patient cohort used in the study. Specific outcomes enable evidence generation associated with the corresponding outcome variables which can be measured in numerous ways.

Formulating a clinical question that is relevant to the PICO is equally important. There are many different methods that can be used to develop a clinical question although many debate around the broadness or narrowness of these. Tables 2.1 and 2.2 demonstrate common clinical questions, outcomes, and outcome measures used in clinical trials and epidemiology studies.

Table 2.1 Common clinical questions, outcomes, and outcome measures for epidemiology studies.

Common epidemiology questions	Common outcomes	Relevant outcome measure
Questions about prevalence	Disease burden	Measure of the disease burden using a validated questionnaire and/or test
Questions about risk of disease	Risk factors	Measure of the risk factors using a validated questionnaire and/or test
Questions about diagnosis	Diagnostic accuracy	Measure of the diagnostic method either with a validation procedure and/or statistical method
Questions about prognosis	Mortality and morbidity	Measure of the prevalence of the reported deaths, incidence, and morbidity
Questions about phenomena	Attitudes, values, perceptions, and experiences	Measure using questionnaires
Questions about symptomatologies	Rate of a symptom and/or group of symptoms	Measure each symptom using validated questionnaires and/or clinical test results
Questions about disease progression	Disease severity	Measure severity based on a scoring systems such as a frailty index, clinical tests, and/or disability status

Table 2.2 Common clinical questions, outcomes, and outcome measures for clinical trials.

Common clinical trials questions	Common outcomes	Relevant outcome measure
Questions about the effectiveness of drugs	Safety, morbidity, and mortality	Pharmacokinetics and Pharmacodynamics evaluations using blood and imaging tests
Questions about the effectiveness of medical devices	Safety, morbidity, and mortality	
Questions about the safety profile of a drug and/or combination drug treatment	Frequency of Serious Adverse Events (SAE), Suspected unexpected serious adverse reaction (SUSAR), or Adverse Events	Number of SAEs, SURSARs, and AEs over the course of each phase of the study for the full duration
Questions about the safety profile of a medical device	Frequency of Serious Adverse Events (SAE), Suspected unexpected serious adverse reaction (SUSAR), or Adverse Events	Number of SAEs, SURSARs, and AEs over the course of the study
Questions about cost-effectiveness	Cost to gain a unit of a health outcome or preventable mortality and incremental clinical benefits	Quality adjusted life-year and ratios of incremental costs
Questions about validity	Overall result of effectiveness and efficacy of the interventions associated within the trial	Measurement of the assessment and criteria of the measurement

Validation

In addition to reporting the outcomes and interpretation of these, validation of the research is an important facet. Within epidemiology studies, validity could diminish due to information bias. Mitigating issues with accuracy of a measure, the use of a control cohort, or the use of cross validation with split-sample approach could ensure the robustness of epidemiology studies.

In the context of clinical trials, clinical and statistical validations are important [2]. Thus, these would be assessed and reported using processes that are directly associated with accuracy and precision of endpoints. Subsequent statistical tests could be used to further validate endpoints consistently such as Pearson's correlation coefficient, Intraclass correlation coefficient, Bradley–Blackwood procedure, Concordance correlation coefficient, and Patient coefficient of variation. Based on these findings, statistical simulation methods could be completed to measure the validation of the endpoints using a linear relationship and/or bias based on the difference of means or variances.

Validation is a key component for novel interventions such as those using Artificial Intelligence (AI) where predicting prognosis or diagnosis of a disease has become a vital tool to assist clinicians. Statistically, these models are referred to as risk models, prognostic or diagnostic prediction models using multivariable regression framework based on risk values or estimates using multiple predictors such as smoking status, biomarkers, and age. Thus, these types of tools require validation at two levels: firstly, at the intervention level which ensures methodological rigour, reproducibility, and performance; and secondly, at a user level with a clinical trial and/or an epidemiology study.

A summary of key validation methods is described in Table 2.3.

Table 2.3 Key validation methods.

Validation method	Description	Examples
Face validity	This is the least scientific method used as this is not statistically quantified but is reported based on subjective judgements	Multiple measurements of instruments; where Quizlet is common. Quizlet measures the perspective of the person taking the test
Content validity	This method checks for the content measures is within the scope of the clinical question. The measure could be considered subjective as perception is taken into consideration. Although content validation can be useful when it can be separated from the target population with the use of robust statistical tests	Commonly used with cohort studies or surveys where the content domain is represented. A structured factor analysis using a specific theoretical factor is common
Construct validity	This demonstrates a collection of behaviours associated with the research purpose, where the research measure remains within this construct. Construct validity also includes convergent validity, discriminative validity, nomological network, and multitriat-multimethod matrix. Convergent validity operates in the same manner as observations or operations that are demonstrated in theory. On the other hand, discriminative validity adequately differentiates in a single or group of factors which does not	Commonly used in mental health studies, for example to report findings of depression. Depression is a construct representing personality traits that is manifested through various behavioural patterns. Construct validation could be evaluated with inferences made through observations or operationalised components

Table 2.3 Key validation methods—cont'd

Validation method	Description	Examples
	differ from theoretical reasons or prior research. Nomological networks represent constructs of interests that are observations within the scope of the research question that could be developed for a measure. On the other hand, multitrate-multimethod matrix takes six considerations that explore the trait methods of unit and multiple methodologies as well as characteristics	
Internal validity	The method refers to extent to the independent variables that could be accurately reported based on the observed effect. Internal validity reports if the research conducted has produced accurate results. There are number of aspects that could improve internal validity of an experiment, such as blinding, randomisation, random selection, simulation, and validated procedures to report accurate measurables. Internal validity could be threatened by issues with attrition, confounding, diffusion, statistical regression and bias, instruments and testing methods	Internal validity is commonly used to establish cause-and-effect between an outcome and a treatment. For example, if a complex intervention as a smoking cessation tool was provided to a cohort of smokers which was then assessed over a period of time to view any improvements. Internal validity calculation in this scenario would be based on the procedures conducted to assess improvement and scientific rigour of this by way of evaluating confounding. The lower the confounding, the higher the internal validity
External validity	This method refers to the generalizability of the results and the degree of generalizability. There are three types of generalizability of population, environment, and temporal. External validation could be threatened with pre and postprocedural events or effects, characteristics of the sample, selection bias, and situational factors	External validity focuses on the application in the real-world. For example, reprocessing or calibration of the gathered data using statistical methods could adjust any issues with key characteristics such as age, weight or height. This could also be completed using different samples and conducted a metaanalysis that could determine the effect size using independent variables. For metaanalysis using individual participant data, external validation is important, especially if the outcome is associated with clinical prediction models. These could also include combined datasets where the methodological challenges and reporting issues are foreseen as common problems to a novel method of using data

Continued

Table 2.3 Key validation methods—cont'd

Validation method	Description	Examples
Statistical conclusion validity	This method determines the relationship between the effect variables and cause. This method is suitable for reliable procedural measures and adequate sampling methods where the *P*-values demonstrate credibility. Statistical conclusion validity could be effected by low statistical power due to small sample sizes, issues with internal validity, and heterogeneity as well as unreliability of measures	Commonly used in clinical trials with investigational medicinal products such as combination therapy use in cancers versus conventional treatment methods as chemotherapy
Criterion-related validity	This is also referred to as instrumental validity that is measured the quality of the measure. The accuracy of the measurement is compared with an accepted standard. The criterion measured here includes a standard judgement which included predictive and concurrent validity. Predictive validity operationalises predictability based on theory. The measures predict anticipated outcomes. On the other hand, concurrent validation operationalises the ability to determine between theory and reality where the test correlate to measures that may be validated as part of prior research	Commonly used to test performance in different ways. For example, psychometric research, the construct of the test or operationalisation of the test would be assessed with the assistance of theoretical frameworks

2.2 Clinical trials

Pilot study

High-quality outcomes can be secured with an initial *pilot* study to obtain initial outcomes to assess the feasibility of performing a larger-scale clinical trial that has an experimental design and accurate performance. The research protocol associated with a pilot study allows for better planning and modifications to be made that could improve both the operational management and scientific validity. This includes any recruitment and retention issues as well as procedures required for the study. In addition, a pilot study could assess randomisation and blinding methods used, as well as detailed procedures for preparation, storage, and delivery. Acceptability of the intervention to a patient is an important facet assessed in the pilot study.

Phase I

Phase I clinical trials assess the toxicity profile to define a drug dose that is suitable for assessing granular details of pharmacokinetics and pharmacodynamics. Phase IIa clinical trials characterise the drug profile assessing the efficacy as the primary endpoint. Traditionally maximum tolerated dose (MTD) of drugs was tested in Phase I although now this is considered as Phase Ib or Phase IIa. This flexibility is quite useful to assess a diverse array of drugs including combination treatments. Dose–response evaluations and any potential plateau as well as minimally effective doses could be reported more effectively with flexible trial designs.

Phase II

Phase II trials are considered as those conducted to explore therapeutic efficacy and in drug trials, assess the pharmacokinetics (PK) and pharmacodynamics (PD) to develop a PK/PD model and thereby a relevant safety profile by way of evaluating adverse reactions. Additionally, preliminary evidence of the drug profile would be reported with efficacy as a primary endpoint. Often phase II trial publications could compare combination treatments versus a single regimen and/or routine treatment versus the trial drug. The design associated with Phase II clinical trials would enable assessment of key questions to plan for Phase III.

Phase III

Phase III trials are conducted to determine optimal doses to be provided at safe level of, frequency of dosing, and administration routes. Therefore, this phase provides a therapeutic confirmatory or comparative efficacy endpoint. As a result, Phase III is referred to as placebo-controlled or superiority trial that compares interventions relatively easily. Phase II and Phase III can be intertwined in some instances, and it is not uncommon to have similar or vastly different findings. There is an argument for a placebo effect and variations including unexpected improvements on acute symptoms which could be seen to regress to the mean as the study continues. Hence, the application of placebos including surgical placebos has been debated in line with the Declaration of Helsinki. This stage of the clinical development pathway comprises a large sample size and a more rigorous assessment of common and uncommon adverse reactions.

Phase IV

Drug side effects (DSEs) are a major health problem around the world. In the United States alone, for example, they have been responsible for over 2 million hospitalisations each year. DSEs represent a financial burden to developed countries [3], since they are associated with large sums spent every year.

Phase IV trials are a crucial part of the postmarketing stage for drug trials. Historically, medical device trials move into Phase IV relatively quickly in comparison to drug trials. However, this has changed with the evolving scientific and regulatory landscape. In the United Kingdom, drugs and medical devices are rigorously overseen to assess cost-effectiveness and deliverability within the NHS. In addition, during Phase IV, a wider consensus to long-term side effects and/or adverse reactions is reviewed. In some instances, long-term effects may not have been detected in the previous three steps, which are always constrained by both time and number of participants.

Although premarketing studies and analyses are rigorous and mandatory for all new drugs, the safety profile of a drug at the time of regulatory approval is often inefficient. This occurs due to certain characteristics of phase I–III studies, such as limited sample size, short-term studies, and lack of well-defined inclusion/exclusion criteria.

Phase IV trials, also known as 'therapeutic use' or 'postmarketing' studies, include observational studies performed with drugs approved by regulatory agencies to identify possible and less common side effects and assess costs and actual effectiveness of the drug in similar diseases, populations, or doses in populations other than those tested in the study [HF1].

Phase IV clinical trials differ significantly from earlier phases in their study design, requirements, and scientific demands. Phases I through III primarily examine the drug's safety profile on a smaller scale, as well as the drug's effectiveness in a controlled setting of a randomised clinical trial (RCT). One of the main objectives of phase IV studies is to detect flaws in the pharmacovigilance of a drug, in addition to being able to perform analyses with a larger sample of the previous phases (I–III) [4]. Pharmacovigilance activities are 'assessment and prevention of dangerous drugs or any other problems related to detection, evaluation, prevention of dangerous drugs, or any other problem' [5] and play a crucial role in making sure that patients receive safe drugs, also minimising side effects.

There are several types of studies that can be part of a phase IV trial, such as observational studies, standard randomised clinical trials, drug interaction studies, or special populations. An important feature of these studies is that they are generally larger with a more diverse and heterogeneous population than in preclinical studies. In addition, the study scenario aims to resemble real-world conditions [4]. The safety and diligence of postmarketing trials go far beyond Phases I–III. Phase IV trials address, for example, long-term safety, patient participation, and budget. These points are of utmost importance to regulatory agencies, but also to other stakeholders, such as physicians, sponsors, and patients. In contrast to phase-III trials, which usually approach a single study design, phase IV requires several types of design [4].

The purpose of this section is to elucidate the different study approaches that are relevant in phase IV. The latter involves a wide range of study designs, all of these with advantages and disadvantages. Therefore, we cannot say that one is better than the other. However, to reach a high level of validity and reliability, it is extremely important for researchers to choose the correct methodology for their specific study [6].

Postmarketing surveillance studies

The focus of this type of study is to identify possible adverse drug reactions and ensure efficient monitoring of the drug after it has been launched on the market. It is an adjunct to spontaneous monitoring systems. Besides, it is intended to detect failures that may signal the existence of a problem [7]. Adverse drug reactions that may occur in patients during phases I–III are unlikely to be detected during these phases. Moreover, they may not yet be known at the time a drug is approved by the regulatory agencies. These adverse reactions are rare (fewer than 1 in 3000–5000) and are more likely to be detected when large numbers of patients are exposed to a drug after its approval and commercialisation [8].

Endpoints and surrogate endpoints

Nowadays, the creation of a new drug is surrounded by huge challenges, for example, the correct response of the drug in the population sample; and slow and expensive clinical development processes, which are often inefficient. A very important point that influences the duration and complexity of this process is the choice of parameter(s) to be used to assess and quantify the effectiveness of the new drug [9].

Clinically relevant outcomes are often difficult to use in research. This can happen when: (1) the equipment used to assess the impact of a disease is expensive. This is the the case of cachexia, which is a disease that causes loss of muscle tissue associated with malnutrition and whose equipment used to assess nitrogen, potassium levels, and water in the patients' bodies, often makes the experiment financially unfeasible. It can also occur when: (2) there is difficulty in measuring the data; for example, quality-of-life assessments that involve multidimensional instruments that are difficult to validate, and (3) large samples due to the low incidence of the event of interest; for example, cytotoxic drugs can have serious, though rare, side effects, such as leukaemia induced by topoisomerase inhibitors. One way to solve this problem is to opt for cheaper, more frequently used, or more conventional endpoints.

Surrogate endpoints have been used in medical research for a long time. Despite the potential advantages of surrogate endpoints, their use has been surrounded by controversy. We can use as an example the case in which the Food and Drug Administration (FDA), in 1994, approved three antiarrhythmic drugs (encainide, flecainide, and moricizine), based only on the main effects, which were to decrease arrhythmia episodes [9]. It was believed that by decreasing and controlling arrhythmia episodes, the mortality rate of patients with heart disease would also decrease, since at the time it was proven that the mortality rate for arrhythmic patients was four times higher. However, after the marketing period, it was found that the mortality rate of these drugs was twice that of the placebo group [10].

An endpoint represents the clinical status or health status of a patient who has undergone research. It aims to assess the benefits or damages of a treatment. A clinical outcome describes a valid measure of clinical benefit from treatment, i.e. the impact of treatment on how a patient feels, functions, and survives [HF2] [11]. The endpoints can also be divided into two steps: primary endpoints are used to accurately calculate the sample size to be used in the research, as well as to judge and evaluate the effectiveness of the study once completed. In a complementary way, secondary endpoints help to assess the therapeutic efficiency of a given study, but they do not have enough power to assess whether the results are positive or not [HF3] [12].

A surrogate endpoint is a clinical trial result used as an alternative for a direct measure of how a patient will respond to a particular intervention and whether that intervention has worked. A surrogate endpoint does not have the ability to directly measure the primary clinical benefit, but it is expected that it can directly contribute to identifying whether there was a benefit in the tested population. In general, predictive nature of a surrogate outcome is determined by evaluating epidemiological, therapeutic, pathophysiological, or other scientific evidence [HF4] [13].

Surrogate outcomes are used because they can be measured earlier, are usually convenient or less invasive, and can accelerate the approval process of a new technique, a new drug, or a new material. Furthermore, there are other advantages such as reduce the sample size of clinical trials and decrease the duration of the study, thus reducing the total cost of the experiment [HF5] [14]. A surrogate endpoint basically is an endpoint that is intended to replace clinical endpoint of interest that cannot be observed in a trial [HF6].

Endpoint surrogates may override clinical outcomes in some trials. For example, surrogate endpoints are used when clinical outcomes, such as stroke, may take a long time to study. They are also used in cases where conducting a clinical outcome study would be unethical. Before a surrogate outcome can be accepted in lieu of a clinical outcome, extensive evidence must be accumulated, including evidence from epidemiological studies and clinical trials [15].

When a surrogate outcome predicts a beneficial effect through appropriate studies, its use often allows for more efficient drug development programmes. For example, many clinical trials use a variety of drugs to control blood pressure. These drugs demonstrate that lowering systolic blood pressure reduces the risk of a stroke. Thus, the reduction measurement in the surrogate endpoint of systolic blood pressure can be substituted with the clinical outcome of stroke. Clinical trials aimed at reducing the risk of a stroke can be conducted more rapidly in smaller populations using the validated surrogate endpoint.

Clinical trial designs

Current paradigms assess incremental clinical benefits between multiple treatments that have either same or comparable response kinetics. Trial designs have evolved over the past few decades, especially from a scientific perspective. Modern-day designs promptly attempt to use more flexible design methods to obtain data more efficiently, rapidly, and in a cost-effective manner, especially since each disease area and treatment intervention will have their own challenges.

Adaptive design

Adaptive study designs are flexible in comparison to most of clinical trial practices as they add a linear-process driven approach with an analysis sequence. It is common practice to review the data as part of an interim analysis whilst the trial is ongoing. The validity and integrity of the trial remain the same

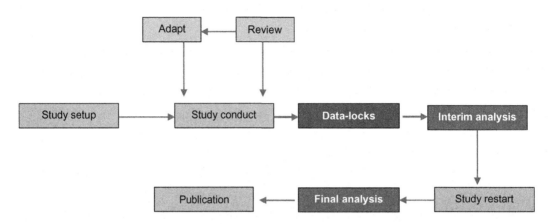

Fig. 2.1 Adaptive study design framework.

as the data accumulation remains specific to a particular time-frame for the purpose of the interim analysis (Fig. 2.1).

Adaptive designs permit refining sample sizes, allocation ratios to different arms, and participant identification. Multiple adaptations could be used in a single trial, for example, a sequential design could be used for revising sample size estimation and/or randomisation. Adaptive clinical trials could also be used across the phases of I, II, and III. More specific examples are demonstrated in Table 2.4.

The practicality of conducting an adaptive clinical trial is seldom discussed despite the importance of understanding the differences when comparing to a traditional fixed design. Additional considerations such as drug or medical device supply are important to ensure that there are imbalances in recruitment in multi-centre trials. For trials with a ratio allocation where multiple treatments are available to participants, changes to these can be made after the trial commences. Thus, in these instances, a centralised randomisation system should be used to ensure minimising errors. Drug or medical device supply chains mostly use centralised methods such as this to ensure dispensing records could be equally overseen.

Analysing data in adaptive designs is different in comparison to most traditional trial data. Many adaptive clinical trials can use multiple hypotheses such as the MAMS trials, in addition to re-testing the same hypothesis multiple times with the use of effects on multiple trial endpoints sequentially. These could lead to an increase in type I error rates. Type I error rates could be managed at a fixed level with adjustments made during the analysis at multiple timepoints using linear methods. For example, in the

Table 2.4 Examples of clinical trials.

Design	Methodology/overview of the design	Examples of clinical trials
Sequential	Sequential analyses where statistical procedures could be calculated at any stage of the study prior to the end. A sequential design could have efficacy, futility or safety as a measure to define early termination of the trial	DEVELOP-UK
Multiarm multistage	Exploration of multiple doses of the same drug or multiple treatments could be used in the same trial. Combinational therapies could also be used to review early efficacy and remove any of those that have a suboptimal clinical performance based on the chosen outcome measures	STAMPEDE, 18-F PET study, COMPARE
Sample size re-estimation	Unblinded or blinded based sample size re-estimation differs based on two concepts' conditional power and group sequential trials. In the instance of conditional power which is a futility test to remain flexible	DEVELOP-UK
Adaptive dose-escalation	Allocation ratios could be adjusted to inform doses and drug profiles	DILfrequency
Adaptive randomisation	Allocation ratio could be adjusted towards the optimal treatment	DexFEM
Population enrichment	Specific recruitment methods where patients are aligned to the treatment from a variety of ethnicities and races	Rizatriptan study
Seamless transition from phase I/II	Combining activity and safety of the intervention into a single study	MK-0572, MATCHPOINT
Seamless transition from phase II/III	Combining a section of confirmatory steps into a single study	PIVOTAL
Adaptive biomarkers	Adapt biomarkers as outcomes measures at various stages	FOCUS 4, DIL Frequency
Continuous assessment and/or reassessment	Dose escalation using a model to estimate a maximum tolerated dose	TRAFIC, RomiCar

MAMS trials, adjustments were made to maintain varying doses or regimens of the same intervention. However, this method would be unnecessary in the event there are multiple interventions across multiple patient cohorts within the same adaptive clinical trial. Thus, adjusting for multiplicity requires careful understanding of the data and logical consistency with data of an equivalent trial with two arms. Another facet to consider in this scenario would be the regulatory guidelines associated with adjusting multiple tests within a single trial, unless it is considered as a combinational-treatment setting. Statistical software packages catered to adaptive trials are commercially available to ensure that quality control steps could be used to complete accurate data analysis (Table 2.5).

Table 2.5 Examples of statistical analyses packages.

Statistical output	Traditional, fixed clinical trial	Adaptive clinical trial	Solution	Example of software package
Sample size				Statsol
Effect estimate	Unbiased across many trials where the mean is reported as a true measure	Treatment effects are estimated therefore reported figures could be bias with an incorrect mean value	Adjusted estimators could minimise bias	Adoptr package
			Statistical simulation could be explored the level of bias followed by a sensitivity analysis	Adoptr package
P-Value	Calibrated with nominal significance which could also be considered to the type I error rate	Traditional P-value calculations may be conservative	Theoretical calibration of the P-value would be useful as combining data from different stages will require an inverse of the normal method	AdpatTest, ADDPLAN, OptGS
			Statistical simulation to explore type I error design	AdpatTest, ADDPLAN, OptGS
Confidence interval	95% confidence intervals demonstrate a true effect	Computed confidence intervals could be incorrect	Use a coverage level to report confidence intervals	Adoptr package
			Use statistical simulation to report actual coverage	Adoptr package
Subgroup analysis				Adoptr package
Direct variation		Variational problems associated with dual stage sample size functions	Use of Gaussian quadrature rule of degree k	Adoptr package

Interpretability of trial results could be challenging due to the manner in which triallists design and conduct adaptive trials. For example, the use of interim data to modify trials could raise operational bias that is often not addressed in publications. Interim results could also lead to speculation or knowledge bias once the data-locks are released and the study recommences, in particular amongst the investigative team and the scientific community. As such, access to interim data should be minimised even within the trialist team until the study has ended, with strict confidentiality maintained with the help of a Quality Assurance team [16,17], with specific models for monitoring using risk-based approaches than conventional methods. This could also minimise potential inconsistencies with study delivery, at different stages and improve the credibility of the trial findings. For example, if the eligibility criteria are altered leading to a change in the patient population, results may show a shift before and after this change was made, and further complicate trial findings if compared to interim analysis results. Therefore, ensuring all publications address such factors within the strengths and limitations section could assist with maintaining both internal and external validity. Modifications do not equally prevent a combined-results section to demonstrate overall treatment effects. Adding a subgroup analysis by geographical location could further minimise any overrepresentation of the findings, whilst still maintaining the integrity associated with generalisability of trial findings.

Platform design [18–21]

Platform trials are commonly used to assess multiple interventions simultaneously and comparing to a common control group using a master protocol. The platform design is an extension of adaptive designs, often referred as a multistage design, arm, and intervention method using a multiinterim evaluation map. The level of flexibility in platform trials has allowed novel experimental arms to be added and compared to the same control arm patients during the course of the trials, whilst the same operational infrastructure and standardisation of procedures remain (Fig. 2.2).

Fig. 2.2 demonstrates the addition of different interventions where the ability to close-an intervention arm, whilst adding a new interventional arm flexibly, without stopping the overall study.

Platform trials also offer an advantage to traditional design by way of having disease-focused approaches rather than intervention-focused, where the assessment of interventions is able to efficiently

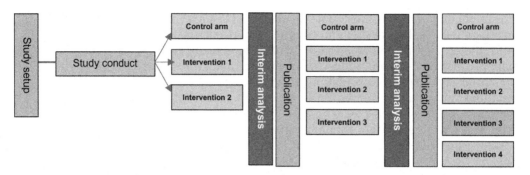

Fig. 2.2 Platform design framework.

report effectiveness yields. Disease focus means most platform trials will have a research question around the most suited intervention that will benefit a patient in comparison to a placebo or a gold standard. Platform data collection methods are nonstandardised given the design of the multiarm and multiinterim analysis approach. In many respects, therapeutic discovery moves forward with the advancements in the regulatory landscape, as such, there is a requirement for additional resources, funding, and managing time delays. Platform trials provide the opportunity for regulators, clinical researchers, patients, and policy-makers to work cohesively using a single approach with nomenclature documents for a group of interventions. An example of this type of approach is the RECOVERY or PRINCIPLE or PANORAMIC clinical trials led by the University of Oxford. These approaches have led to a transformation in clinical trial management and other stakeholder involvement to efficiently manage resources and reporting findings more quickly than previously conducted. With growing popularity for platform trials, fundamental principles should become available to all Clinical Trialists. As such, important components that could be explored using a platform design that clinical researchers should consider are demonstrated in Table 2.6.

Basket design

Basket trials are a novel design primarily used in oncology-based targeted therapies to assess a single or combination regimen suited to be directed at one or more targets (Table 2.7). Conceptually, this trial design is associated with precision medicine techniques where biomarkers are commonly used to guide the pharmacokinetics and pharmacovigilance of the treatments provided. Similar to platform trials, basket trials also use a single

Table 2.6 Key clinical components of platform trials.

Aim	Factors required	Key features
Compare interventions	Statistical analysis	Interventions compared with a control
		Comparison of multiple interventions
		The presence/absence of a subgroup effect
	Intervention versus control group	Efficacy of interventions associated with simultaneous activation
		Concurrent control or past control
	Allocation	Allocation ratios between the arms associated within the trial
Interim assessments	Frequency of an interim analysis	Interim assessment
	Interim analysis outcomes	Outcomes within the interim and final analysis should be reported
	Timeframes for interim assessments	Pre and postevaluation period
	Statistical features	Criteria for inclusion and exclusion of an intervention arm
New interventions	Scientific justification for use of a new intervention	Scientific rationale should be used to design the data collection method
	Timeframes for addition of novel interventions	Specific timeframes for novel intervention addition should be included in the statistical analysis
	Mechanism and process for adding a new interventional arm	Scientific and clinical justification for adding the interventions
Recruitment targets for each arm	Variability of recruitment over time	No fixed sample design should be used

master protocol. The frequency of this design has considerably increased with the implementation of immunotherapies over the last decade. Basket trial methodologies could be used to test any molecular therapy regardless of the organ or pathology involved as the data collection could provide insights to predictive responses related to the molecular mechanisms as well as any homogeneous effects associated with different tumour types. Therefore, these trials are beneficial for developing molecular profiles of an array of diseases and not just cancer.

Most basket trials have been used with a noncomparative design aimed to identify populations where the antitumour activity is of more value where the rate of response is assessed as an intermediate primary endpoint. The control group should be

Table 2.7 Methods required to achieve goals of basket trials.

Aim	Factors required	Key features
Compare cohorts with a targeted therapy	Statistical analysis	An indirect comparison
		Stratification per cohort
		Intention to treat analysis
		Clinically relevant endpoints of overall survival, rate of response and quality of life
		Heterogeneity of results evaluation
Recruitment targets for each arm	Comparators use	Minimum of 30 patients should be used across each cohort
Generic target	Biomarker detection	Confirm the prognostic value of any genetic alterations detected
		Combined assessment of the reliability, availability and performance of the diagnostic test
Nested method use	Mortality reported as a primary endpoint	Complete a nested analysis

adapted to the multiple cohorts in the trial based on tumour location, stage, and histology markers. Implementation of a comparative assessment of novel therapies is important both from safety, prognostic value, and efficacy standpoint, as well as increases the risk of bias. Agnostic indications are a possibility and the objective in such instances should be to use the complete sample size to complete a statistical analysis. This type of analysis is not uncommon where the hypothesis of homogeneity across all cohorts is assumed. A subsequent heterogeneity assessment between cohorts should be considered using a systematic approach to report effect size per cohort with an overall estimate using a forest plot. Hence, there are multiple scientifically important issues around data interpretation and clinical challenges around these appear to be a common feature. Operational requirements for basket trials are complex and the use of a single screening platform could be useful. Centralised decision-making pathways are important for adapting elements that require real-time assessments and rapid responses to the data collection. The use of a master protocol within this study design is useful to maintain a steady workflow.

Fig. 2.3 demonstrates the basket trial design and process of conduct. The cohorts used within these trials decided during the study setup stage using preliminary clinical data that shows

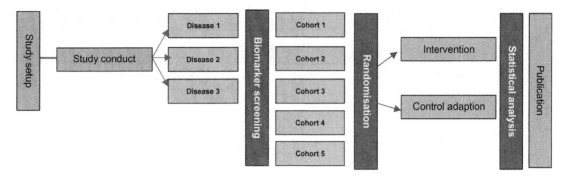

Fig. 2.3 Basket trial design.

evidence of a relationship between the molecular mechanism and preclinical data of antitumour benefit.

2.3 Epidemiology

Lilienfeld in 1978 published a manuscript in which he elucidated some definitions of epidemiology. At the time, there was no consensus amongst epidemiologists regarding the definition of epidemiology. His research goal was to develop a single, clear, and understandable definition of epidemiology that could understand all types of diseases and populations [22]. Lilienfeld based his work on 23 existing definitions of epidemiology and proposed the following definition [23]: 'Epidemiology is a method of reasoning about disease that deals with biological inference derived from observations of disease phenomena in population groups.'

Epidemiology is concerned not only with tracking and defining disease distribution patterns, but also with the factors that influence these patterns. These investigations are usually conducted within a conceptual model or philosophical framework. Thus, epidemiology can be seen as an eclectic integrative discipline that draws strength from diverse disciplines such as biology, ethics, biostatistics, economics, genetics, medicine, psychology, and sociology [24–26] (Fig. 2.4).

Retrospective studies

Retrospective studies use existing data from electronic healthcare systems and/or research data bases that are subtype of Epidemiology. These studies are less expensive and faster to complete where sufficient baseline measurements are available. However, the data used within these studies often are limited and

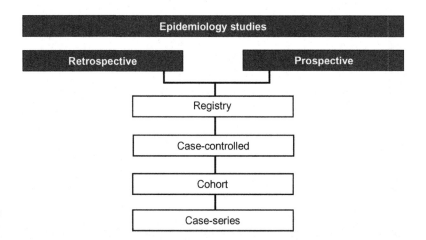

Fig. 2.4 Types of investigation in epidemiology studies.

inconsistent. For example, the quality and nature of the data gathered could differ widely within healthcare systems [27], primary and/or availability of historical data as GDPR or opt-out schemes could mean the legal basis could introduce limitations for the utility of the data.

Retrospective studies could also be conducted at a population level, which are considered ecological studies. These report differences in outcomes between populations or change in population characteristics over a specific timeframe. These are used commonly in women's health to deter causal links to explore alternatives with further investigations at an individual level [28].

Prospective studies

Cross-sectional studies

Cross-sectional studies are defined by disease definitions, risk factors, or symptoms identified during a specific timeframe. These are commonly used to report prevalence across an array of clinical conditions. Table 2.8 explores components of various study types as discussed below.

These could be categorised to either descriptive or analytical by design. Descriptive cross-sectional designs are primarily surveys that assess burden of a disease within a well-defined population. Analytical studies could investigate associations between health outcomes and putative risk factors. A significant limitation could be the ability to report valid conclusions between risk associations as the outcomes are measured simultaneously. Therefore, it is challenging to determine if the exposure incurred pre or post-disease diagnosis. Theoretically, these are two different designs

Table 2.8 Strengths and limitations of different study types.

Study design	Strengths	Limitations
Comparative studies	Inexpensive to complete	Unable to report individual specific exposure(s) with disease but rather average exposure levels
	Retrospective and prospective data could be sued	Unable to control the effects of confounding
	Multiple populations and/or interventions could be used	
Case report/ case series	Used to report findings in a shorter timescale	Minimal use of statistics
	Useful to devise hypothesis associated with potential risk factors for a disease	Experiences reported has minimal generalisability
	More relevant to clinical practice	Conclusions would require further scientific validation
Cross-sectional	Assess exposures	Disease incidence cannot be reported
	Assess disease status	Predisease exposure is inconclusive
	Provide disease prevalence along with outcomes	
	Provides factors of disease survival and aetiology	
Case-controlled	Inexpensive to conduct	High level of selection and recall bias
	Suitable to assess latent periods of diseases	Exposure and disease relationships are difficult to assess with complicated conditions
	Efficient to assess rare diseases	Inefficient to use rare exposures
	Assess multiple aetiological factors for a specified disease	Inefficient to report incidence rates of disease
Cohort	Efficient for assessing rare exposures	
	Retrospective studies are inexpensive	Prospective studies are expensive and time consuming
	Efficient to assess incidence of disease	Retrospective studies require comprehensive medical records
	Prospective studies report minimal bias in ascertainment of exposure	Long-term follow-up data could impact the validity of the final results
Interventional	Often considered as the gold standard of epidemiological research	Sufficient populations may be challenging to use
	Provides robust cause-effect relationship evidence	Expensive and time consuming

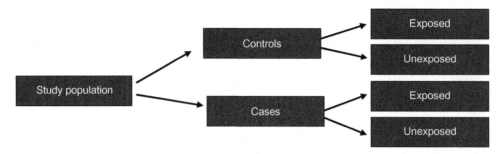

Fig. 2.5 Cross-sectional study design.

but most researchers apply a mixed methods approach especially when reporting epidemics or pandemics in communicable diseases where there are several exposures. The data gathered and analysed from these studies could inform prevalence, coverage, and trends that could represent clinical characteristics that are clinically useful and can be furthered to develop interventions within the research landscape.

Fig. 2.5 show a cross-sectional study which includes exposures, confounders, and outcomes that would be measured simultaneously to report prevalence. Analytical cross-sectional studies could use the same format and use odds ratios to assess the strengths and limitations of risk factors and health outcomes that could be associated with one another.

Case series

Case series studies report observations of a series of individuals that use the same intervention pre and post without the presence of a control group (Fig. 2.6).

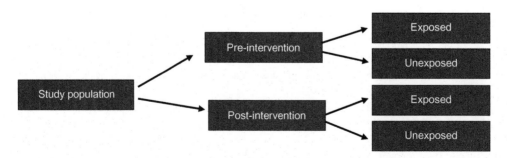

Fig. 2.6 Case study.

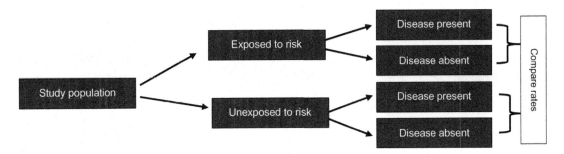

Fig. 2.7 Cohort study.

Cohort studies

Cohort studies evaluate prognosis associated with treatments or aetiologies within a specific timeframe. The most reported cohort studies are that of communicable diseases associated with HIV. In the era of anti-HIV therapy, assessing patterns of treatment efficacy could be easily completed as it contributes significantly to the clinical knowledge base associated with effectiveness, infection incubation periods, and impact of the treatments provided over a period. Cohort studies yield relative risks and incidence rates that may demonstrate unanticipated associations. However, to maximise outputs of a cohort study requires a large sample size and longitudinal datasets albeit this would be expensive. These are also prone to methodological and attrition bias (Fig. 2.7).

Case-controlled studies

Case-controlled studies are explored based on a specific disease or outcome status than an exposure. Case-controlled studies comprise a control and a disease that is able to report frequency (odds) of the exposure. A key feature of the case-controlled study reports statistical inferences between exposure and the disease investigated. An intuitive appeal with these types of studies is its ability to investigate the aetiology. Case-controlled studies could be considered as an extension of a case series and can be expressed relative to people with and without the disease being explored. However, there is a possibility of selection and recall bias. Methodological quality could be improved by way of using conditional logistic regression, odds ratios, confidence intervals for odds ratios, Fisher's extract test, and Chi-square 2 by 2 test (Fig. 2.8).

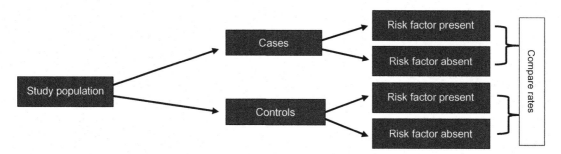

Fig. 2.8 Case-controlled study.

2.4 Epidemiology methodology

The start of any research study would be to develop a relevant question and agree on objective to design the study. Understanding the research goals facilitates the process of reporting the findings. This is a multistaged process. These include identifying the following aspects as part of developing an epidemiology methodology.

The hypotheses and the goals of a study are the keys to determining the study design and statistical tests that are most appropriate to use as illustrated in Table 2.9. Epidemiology studies have a classification scheme that broadly covers descriptive and analytical components (Fig. 2.9). Descriptive epidemiology focuses on incidence and prevalence of diseases by population and locations. Analytical epidemiology comprises aetiology, pathophysiology, and treatments generated from descriptive studies.

Epidemiological statistical methods are driven by evidence-based medicine (EBM); often these could be health-service-based research. These are reported often as healthcare-outcome-based studies.

Table 2.9 Examples of hypotheses.

Key factors	Examples
Develop a hypothesis The aims of the study	What is the efficacy of the drug or medical device under specific conditions
	What is effectiveness of the drug or medical device in population
	What are the causes or risk factors for a disease
	What is the disease burden in the community
	What is the quality of the management of the activity
	What is the cost-effectiveness of a particular treatment or diagnostic tool

Case study

The term 'master protocol' is fairly new within clinical research. The starting point of a master protocol method was part of clinical trials in oncology and haematology primarily, although this has translated to various other interventional studies. A master protocol is a unification of multiple cohorts, drugs, and methods. Effective oncological studies benefit from simultaneously assessing drugs and/or multiple tumour types using a structured approach. Given the regulatory landscape, a single protocol approval would reduce study setup timeframes, costs, and effective use of infrastructure.

The Biomarker-Integrated Approaches of Targeted therapy for Lung Cancer Elimination-1 (BATTLE-1 TRIAL) is a good example of an umbrella trial with four parallel phase II studies for patients that had been treated with chemotherapy and experienced disease relapse. The treatment of the trial targets four genetic pathways where 1:1:1:1 randomisation is used. The outcomes use an adaptive-randomisation scheme where the updated knowledge is used in a *real-time, real-world* setting. Patients receive more efficacious treatments as the trial progresses.

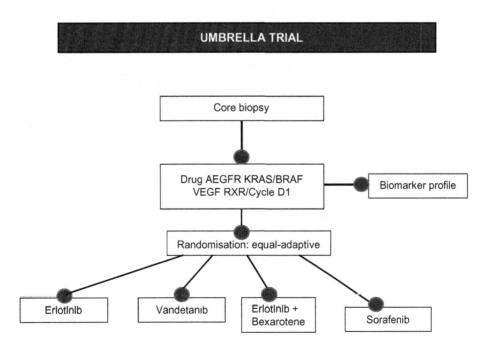

Fig. 2.9 Umbrella trial.

Learning objectives

1. Cost savings have been shown to work well especially at the setup and recruitment stages, ongoing trial monitoring, and administration. Leveraging the same infrastructure, including continuous resource use without any redundancies which largely impact academic trials due to limitations in funding availability.

2. Reducing timeframes to effectively and efficiently assess an intervention is vital as often regulatory and governance approvals could delay study initiation. In addition, reducing lead-up timeframes also shortens the timescales required for licencing and implementation to clinical practice.

3. There are various benefits:

   a. Personalised medicine is the future of clinical medicine and is a more accepted method of clinical treatment for patients. For example, targeted-therapy clinical trials are more accepted by patients in comparison to conventional treatments, especially within the field of oncology. The placebo exposure from a 1:1 ratio to 1:5 could drastically reduce side effect endeavoured by patients. This method could also provide more options to patients that may otherwise be limited.

   b. Researchers benefit from master protocol use as their time is more efficiently used during the study setup and delivery stages. The data collection is more unified using a single protocol approach leading to an easier analysis as the natural history of cohorts assists with confirming clinical hypothesis.

   c. Advocacy groups benefit from master protocols as the preclinical research could be accelerated and recruitment optimised.

4. Continuous improvement, implementation, and dissemination of research evidence for real-world consumption are important. Complex diseases and demands of patients are a growing challenge global healthcare systems are facing. Therefore, learning from clinical research outcomes is a fundamental component to improve diagnosis and treatments.

References

[1] Delanerolle G, Rathod S, Elliot K, Ramakrishnan R, Thayanandan T, Sandle N, et al. Rapid commentary: ethical implications for clinical trialists and patients associated with COVID-19 research. World J Psychiatry 2021;11(3):58–62. https://doi.org/10.5498/wjp.v11.i3.58.

[2] Barnard-Kelly K, Whicher CA, Price HC, Phiri P, Rathod S, Asher C, et al. Liraglutide and the management of overweight and obesity in people with severe mental illness: qualitative sub-study. BMC Psychiatry 2022;22:21. https://doi.org/10.1186/s12888-021-03666-5.

[3] Zhang X, Zhang Y, Ye X, Guo X, Zhang T, He J. Overview of phase IV clinical trials for postmarket drug safety surveillance: a status report from the ClinicalTrials.gov registry. BMJ Open 2016;11(6). https://doi.org/10.1136/bmjopen-2015-010643.

[4] Hadrys A. Phase IV clinical trials. Master's thesis, University of Zagreb; 2021. Retrieved from https://urn.nsk.hr/urn:nbn:hr:105:751986.

[5] Härmark L, Van Grootheest AC. Pharmacovigilance: methods, recent developments and future perspectives [Internet]. Eur J Clin Pharmacol 2008;64:743–52. https://doi.org/10.1007/s00228-008-0475-9.

[6] Jaeger BT, Deshpande R. Choosing a phase IV study design. Pharm Mark; 2003. p. 29–30.

[7] Cvmp TTO, et al. Committee for veterinary medicinal products guideline for the conduct of post-marketing surveillance studies of veterinary medicinal products. Practice; 2000.

[8] Suvarna V. Phase IV of drug development. Perspect Clin Res 2010;1(2):57–60.

[9] Buyse M, Molenberghs G, Paoletti X, Oba K, Alonso A, Van der Elst W, et al. Statistical evaluation of surrogate endpoints with examples from cancer clinical trials. Biom J 2016;58(1):104–32. https://doi.org/10.1002/bimj.201400049.

[10] DeGruttola V, Fleming TR, Lin DY, Coombs R. Validating surrogate markers—are we being naive? J Infect Dis 1997;175:237–46. https://doi.org/10.1093/infdis/175.2.237.

[11] Biomarkers Definitions Working Group. Biomarkers and surrogate endpoints: preferred definitions and conceptual framework. Clin Pharmacol Ther 2001;69(3):89–95. https://doi.org/10.1067/mcp.2001.113989.

[12] Saad ED, Buyse M. Statistical controversies in clinical research: end points other than overall survival are vital for regulatory approval of anticancer agents. Ann Oncol 2016;27(3):373–8. https://doi.org/10.1093/annonc/mdv562.

[13] FDA-NIH Biomarker Working Group. BEST (Biomarkers, EndpointS, and Other Tools) resource [Internet]. Silver Spring, MD: Food and Drug Administration (US); 2016. Glossary. 2016 Jan 28 [Updated 2021 Nov 29]. Available from https://www.ncbi.nlm.nih.gov/books/NBK338448/.

[14] O'Hara ME, Clutton-Brock TH, Green S, Mayhew CA. Endogenous volatile organic compounds in breath and blood of healthy volunteers: examining breath analysis as a surrogate for blood measurements. J Breath Res 2009;3(2):027005. https://doi.org/10.1088/1752-7155/3/2/027005.

[15] US Food and Drugs. Surrogate endpoint resources for drug and biologic development. [Updated 2022 May 4]. Available from: https://www.fda.gov/drugs/development-resources/surrogate-endpoint-resources-drug-and-biologic-development.

[16] Gallo P. Operational challenges in adaptive design implementation. Pharm Stat 2006;5:119–24. https://doi.org/10.1002/pst.221.

[17] Chow SC, Corey R, Lin M. On the independence of data monitoring committee in adaptive design clinical trials. J Biopharm Stat 2012;22:853–67. https://doi.org/10.1080/10543406.2012.676536.

[18] Woodcock J, LaVange LM. Master protocols to study multiple therapies, multiple diseases, or both. N Engl J Med 2017;377:62–70. https://doi.org/10.1056/nejmra1510062.

[19] Siden EG, Park JJ, Zoratti MJ, Dron L, Harari O, Thorlund K, et al. Reporting of master protocols towards a standardized approach: a systematic review. Contemp Clin Trials Commun 2019;15:100406. https://doi.org/10.1016/j.conctc.2019.100406.

[20] Park JJH, Siden R, Zoratti MJ, Dron L, Harari O, Singer J, et al. Systematic review of basket trials, umbrella trials, and platform trials: a landscape analysis of master protocols. Trials 2019;20:572. https://doi.org/10.1186/s13063-019-3664-1.

[21] Berry SM, Connor JT, Lewis RJ. The platform trial: an efficient strategy for evaluating multiple treatments. JAMA 2015;313:1619–20. https://doi.org/10.1001/jama.2015.2316.

[22] Frérot M, Lefebvre A, Aho S, Callier P, Astruc K, Gléié LSA. What is epidemiology? Changing definitions of epidemiology 1978-2017. Plos One 2018;13(12):e0208442. https://doi.org/10.1371/journal.pone.0208442.

[23] Lilienfeld DE. Definitions of epidemiology. Am J Epidemiol 1978;107(2):87–90. https://doi.org/10.1093/oxfordjournals.aje.a112521.

[24] Broadbent A. Philosophy of epidemiology. Springer; 2013.

[25] Amsterdamska O. Demarcating epidemiology. Sci Technol Hum Values 2005;30(1):17–51. https://doi.org/10.1179/2046905514Y.0000000146.

[26] Morabia A. Enigmas of health and disease: how epidemiology helps unravel scientific mysteries. Columbia University Press; 2014.

[27] Delanerolle G. The triple E: equality, equitable health care, and empowerment—are we there yet? Br J Gen Pract 2022;72(717):150–1. https://doi.org/10.3399/bjgp22X718841.

[28] Briggs O, Delanerolle G, Burton R, Shi JQ, Hamoda H, Hapangama DK. The silent epidemic of urogenital atrophy. Br J Gen Pract 2021;71(713):538–9. https://doi.org/10.3399/bjgp21x717725.

3

Principles of medical statistics

Key messages

- Statistical analysis plans should be made available as a core study setup document
- A data management plan should be made available to all researchers within the team
- All clinical researchers should have an understanding of statistics relevant to the research studies they are part of
- Statistical methodology advancement is inevitable; thus, regular training programmes should be made available for all research staff
- Differentiating Epidemiology and Clinical trial statistics are important, although translatability of methods should always be considered and used when suitable
- Synthesising evidence by way of maximising the available data should be considered

3.1   Introduction

The use of medical statistics is a fundamental part of high-quality clinical research that shares a symbiotic relationship (Fig. 3.1). Statistical knowledge is therefore vital for those working in clinical research. There are over thousands of statistical methods available for use in research, although these could be categorised into two primary categories.

In the early 19th century, Eilert Sundt (1817–75) and Theo Logian pioneered scientific papers demonstrating mortality, nutrition, and poverty across Norwegian populations. This is an important reference in Norwegian public health research. Sundt was influenced by European traditions although the aim was to innovate an improved way to report large quantitative data sets. In the first instance, Sundt combined the analyses of quantitative and qualitative data. He then introduced a concept using the laws and regularities of natural sciences to study society. Sundt believed regulatories were not considered to be caused by natural

Clinical Trials and Tribulations. https://doi.org/10.1016/B978-0-12-821787-0.00008-8

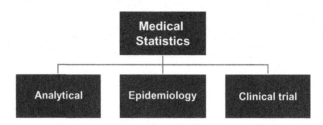

Fig. 3.1 The uses for medical statistics.

conditions that equally impacted individuals as these are prede-termined by birth. The logical basis to Sundt's concept also highlighted that culture, opinions, and societal influences caused certain regularities [1].

Anders Nicolai Kiaer (1838–1919) was the first Director of Statistics in Norway which was an independent entity established in 1876. Kiaer [2] argued that statisticians require nonstatistical knowledge to ensure accurate interpretability.

> 'For that which lies behind the numbers, the pulsating life and the driving forces, is as a rule unintelligible to anyone who does not know and understand the development at close hand so that they are able to explain it', wrote Director Kiær in 1903.

This demonstrated the statistical insight needed to conduct comprehensive epidemiology. The development of the field of epi-demiology also indicated systematic gathering of demographic and economic data. The statistical instruments to diagnose and dissect the details to prescribe treatments were equally demonstrated by the historian Jarin Johannisson. John Graunt (1620–1674), an English Merchant, and William Petty (1623–87), an Economist, Philosopher, and Professor of Anatomy were the first to develop reports about mortality and births, including infant and communicable-disease-based mortality [3]. By way of this exercise, the aim was to prevent diseases and if this was economical for the country. This included the assessment of a per-person cost based on age and gender to demonstrate the impact in society at the time. Another notable book that was of a similar portrayal of epidemiol-ogy was that of Italian physician, Bernardino Ramazzini (1633–1714), *De Morbis Artificum Diatriba (Disease of Workers)* [3]. This book did not show any statistics although the importance of occupational medicine which is based on statistical and epide-miological traditions was discussed, including '*men's diseases*' such as the effects of low morbidity. The book also showed health issues in workplaces as well as potential remedies.

The concept of political arithmetic, which was first introduced in 1749 by German Professor of Philosophy and Law, Gottfried Achenwall (1719–72), was replaced by modern-day statistics. Achenwall demonstrated that political science included social and economic states within the mercantile government ideology. By way of this, early German statisticians emphasised on survival data to contribute to population growth and thereby large, powerful states. However, Sweden was the first to institutionalise statistics by way of the *Tabellverket* or the Census of Sweden in 1749. In a similar manner, Denmark and Norway established the *Rentekammeret* in 1797 [4] which was responsible for finances of the state including advancement of the population demands. The demographic estimates including mortality, life expectancy, and age began to develop leading to the Norwegian Medical Statistics books in the early 19th century. The first step was the preparation and submission of annual health reports across districts and states in 1804 by all Norwegian doctors. The aim of these reports was to provide an overview of disease prevalence, especially scabies, small pox, leprosy, and venereal diseases and mortality amongst infants as well as postnatal mothers. These were referred to in local areas as 'Medicinalberet-ninger' (medical reports) until 1853, it was reported as 'Reports on the State of Health and Medical Conditions in Norway'. These led to the development of the initial health policy efforts in Norway. Historical research sources indicate that Norwegian doctors gathered data on mental illness as well to enable adequate therapy to be provided, including the development of scientific studies. This was argued by the physician Frederik Holst (1791–1871) where three key features should be explored to obtain a census of those with a clinical diagnosis, a classification and diagnostic system, and follow-up of the ill over a period of time. The objective was to study nature of the illness to determine the best way to develop clearer concepts of treatments or a cure [4].

Analytical statistics

Analytical statistics in medicine was developed by French physician Pierre Charles Alexandre Louis (1787–1872) in the 1820s [5]. Louis contributed to the mathematical methods using clinical data from the patients he treated rather than large demographic data. Louis was known for demonstrating that phlebotomy was an unfit method to treat pneumonia. He noted clinical facts, outcomes from autopsies and mortality rates amongst his patients. Based on this data, generalisations were made by Louis to argue a therapeutic method cannot be used without risk, and any effects observed could only be generalised, thus the need for statistics in medical sciences. Louis' work has had a significant impact in mathematical methods in clinical medicine and epidemiology research.

Florence Nightingale (1820–1910) was another personage dedicated to the field of medical statistics by way of using this as a political tool. Nightingale's efforts in establishing modern nursing meant that pioneering efforts had to be made to develop hospital architecture and hospital reform to better measure public health [6]. The first statistical surveys were developed by Nightingale to show that high mortality in hospitals was due to poor hygiene and lack of hierarchical structure to oversee hospital administrations. She developed visual aids such as maps and diagrams which are seen as data charts which are used to report epidemiology studies and clinical trials in the modern era.

Meteorological statistics

The third area of medical statistics developed in the 1840s was medical meteorology which explored the relationship between climate and outbreak of diseases [7]. Details associated with meteorological statistics date back to the Hippocratic text. With frequent epidemic outbreak of diseases, meteorological statistics became important. In the 1840–50s, Danish medicine showed an inclination to study the relationship between climate and disease using large numerical data sets. These analyses were based on the French statistical theory. The Danes used various surveys although there was a lack of evidence to fundamentally explain the mechanistic nature in epidemic theory. Other theories began to rise over the 1860s, which led to the clear modern-day evidence that demonstrates a relationship between climate and seasonable influenza.

3.2   An overview of statistical methods

Statistics are an integral part of clinical research and are driven by the research question, study design, and type of data gathered. Conceptualising statistics in the context of the study is important to ensure that the interpretation and integrity of the data reported remain accurate. Statistics in clinical research primarily comprises of two paradigms: Frequentist and Bayesian (Fig. 3.2). The word paradigm is a recognised scientific method to provide solutions to model problems. The contextual nature of paradigms could depend upon the scientific hypothesis. In terms of statistics, scientific paradigms demonstrate the current state of theories associated with evaluating the data gathered and statistical inference.

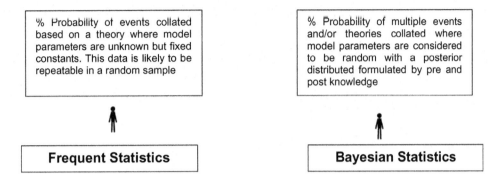

Fig. 3.2 How frequent and Bayesian paradigms are associated with statistics.

Frequentist method

The frequentist method is considered as a traditional statistical inference method to analyse data in a random sample where the probability distributions are based on parameters of θ, *where the inferences are solely driven by a sample. This approach to inference is driven by sample distribution, and the interpretation of this requires a thorough understanding of all inferential procedures. Pragmatically, this could be challenging to translate to real-world scenarios. For instance, a known variance in a sample, a 95% confidence interval population mean μ could have an interval of* $\overline{X} - 1.96\sigma/n, \overline{X} + 1.96\sigma/n.$

Bayesian method

Bayesian theory demonstrates the inverse probability published by Thomas Bayes in 1763 which remains central to the Bayesian paradigm. The Bayesian paradigm relies on the interpretation of probability as a rational conditional measure of uncertainty where it models judgements and their implications. Bayesian methods are based on the axiomatic system which includes initial data to resolve challenges associated with the frequentist methods and thereby explicitly subjective. In contrast to other statistical methods, Bayesian methods use previous knowledge to update beliefs about the likelihood of an event occurring. Based on fresh evidence, this prior knowledge is utilised to adjust the probabilities of an event occurring. This is in contrast to other statistical methods that male inferences only from data. Furthermore, Bayesian approaches express uncertainty using probability distributions, whereas other statistical methods utilise point estimates [8,9]. Specific statistical items are required to report inference using a Bayesian method including prior distribution. Prior distribution can be used as in a graphing format and also by calculating an effective sample size [10]. Conjugate priors are another component that could help solve posterior distributions without complex integrations [10]. The prior function derived mathematically assumes a model based on reports of scientifically justifiable and clinically relevant decisions, leading to objective Bayesian methods. This is increasingly used in *real-world* data-based research.

Bayesian inference is an important analytical method enabling the use of multivariate models using both statistical and machine learning techniques [11]. The sophisticated multivariate models are suitable for complex data sets especially where the data structure and parameters report the outcomes.

The Bayesian research cycle

See Fig. 3.3 and Table 3.1

Empirical Bayes

Empirical Bayes (EB) methods are another important method where the data are used to estimate the unknown on prior and conditional distribution. EB predicators have useful statistical properties including the presence of a linear unbiased predictor (BLUP). Clayton and colleagues explored spatial disease patters using EB [12,13]. A strong criticism of EB models is against uncertainty measures due to the additional variability observed when estimating parameter values that lead to minimal variance [14]. However, variance estimates can be adjusted using other Bayesian methods where underlying rates could be represented.

To make inferences about any unknown parameters, a model will need to be developed using the Bayes' rule. Unknown parameters θ from data (O) could use the following [14,15]:

A model $f(O|\theta)$ demonstrates likelihood.

A prior distribution of θ is calculated before preparing the data.

The likelihood and prior distribution are combined by Bayes' rule to lead to a posterior distribution equation as follows:

$$\text{Posterior } \alpha \text{ Prior} \times \text{Likelihood}$$

Fully Bayesian

In the presence of unknown parameters in priors, EB can have a point estimate where a fully Bayesian model could lead to prior distributions being placed against any unknown parameters. A few parameters result in a hierarchical model structure with

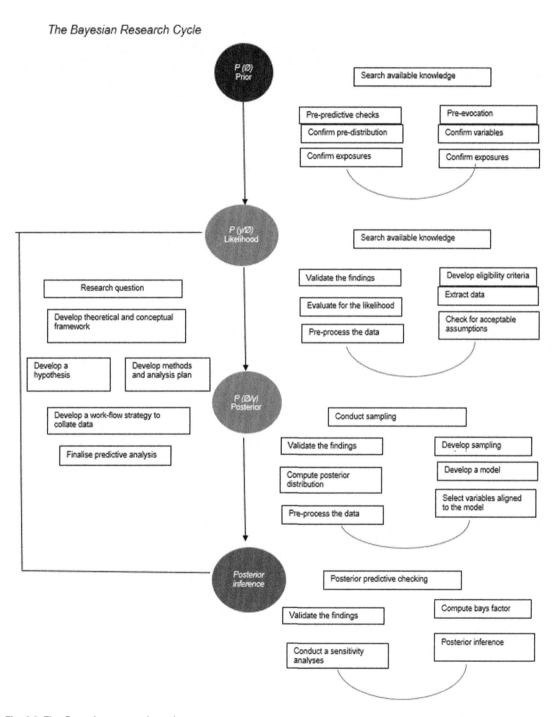

Fig. 3.3 The Bayesian research cycle.

Table 3.1 The advantages and disadvantages of statistical measures.

Statistical measure	Advantage	Disadvantage
Mean	Efficient to use as a test of statistical significance and subsequent analysis	Sensitive to extreme outliers with small sample sizes
	Simplest average to report and understand	Ineffective as a central tendency measure as it skews distribution of data
	Quickest to compute	Ineffective to report nominal or nonnominal ordinal data
Median	Not distorted by outliers and can be deduced for an ordinal scale, ratio, and interval	Inefficient for use of individual time point assessments
	Efficient informative descriptive measure	
Mode	Effective measure to report possible aetiology of disease	Less amenable than the median
	Useful for qualitative data	Potential factor for misinterpretation as a bimodal factor
	Time efficient to understand and calculate	Unstable for data sets with small values
	Effective with extreme values	Not well defined
	Easy identifier in a discrete frequency distribution	
Range	Simple to calculate	Unstable estimate as the number increases with sample size
	Rigidly defined	Lacks the use of all observations and therefore interpretation could be difficult
Variance	Effective to report all deviations from the mean	Sensitive to outliers
	Summarise individual observations with the mean	
Standard deviation	Data dissemination is precise	Difficult to interpret
	Clustered data around the mean is demonstrated	Difficult to calculate
	Effective to further algebraic treatment	Impacted by outliers
	Minimal affects due to fluctuations in a sample	Impacted by extreme values
Coefficient of variation	Ineffective when comparing 2 or more distributions	Lacks variability when the mean changes
	Unitless and applicable to any quantifiable data	Susceptible to changes if the mean varies
	Efficient for comparing unrelated entities	Ineffective to be used to report intervals of the mean
Standard error of mean	Effective to compare means of differing populations	Misinterpretation is common when substituted for SD
	Efficient to demonstrate intervals within population mean	Misinterpretation is common if used to discuss increased precision of the data
Correlation coefficient	Effectively shows the presence or absence of two variables in a single relationship	Specific to correlation research only
	Quantitative data can be analysed easily	Inconclusive to report the reason for the presence or absence of a relationship

multilevels defining the observed data and unknown parameter relationship. The most common use of a Bayesian hierarchical [16] model for the purpose of disease mapping is the BYM model which furthered Clayton and Kaldor's model where a key characteristic is the use of two random effects: one with a spatial structured approach and the other an unstructured [17–19].

The BYM model could be expressed using the following equation:

$$O_i \sim \text{Poisson } (E_i\theta_i)$$

$$\text{Log } (\theta_i) = \alpha + u_i + v_i$$

where

O_i demonstrates the disease events in the ith region

E_i indicates the anticipated case numbers

θ_i shows the incidence ratio

α is referred to as the intercept

The formula indicates an extra-Poisson variability with the inclusion of two spatial random effects of v_i demonstrating inter-area heterogeneity, and u_i indicates spatial components [20,21]. An alternative approach would be to use the *Leroux prior* [22] with the following equation:

Instead of $u_i + v_i$ of the BYM model, the Leroux prior comprises a multivariate normal prior:

$$\mathbf{b} \sim \text{Normal}_I \left(\mathbf{0}, \sum\nolimits_b\right)$$

$$\frac{1}{\sum_b} = \frac{1}{\delta_{b^2}}\left(\lambda(\mathbf{D}_u - \mathbf{W}) + (1 - \lambda)\mathbf{I}_I\right)$$

$\lambda = 0$ and 1 indicating spatial correlation parameter that represents the proportion of excess Poisson variation described spatial dependencies

$D =$ represents a diagonal matrix with $\mathbf{D}_{ii} = \mathbf{n}_i$

$W =$ spatial weight matrix

$I =$ identity matrix

Probabilistic diagnosis

'Probability' is defined in different mannerisms although in Bayesian statistics, this would be a conditional measure of uncertainty that is associated with an event which is an accepted assumption [21]. Thus, probability as a measure could be rationalised as events under conditions where uncertainty is measured along with the conditions under which events take place. Therefore, probabilities are not absolute.

This could be further delineated by assessing probability of an event using available data, a set of assumptions associated with generating the data, as well as the knowledge used to develop the assumptions. These two concepts could be demonstrated mathematically as below:

$$P = \frac{E}{C} \text{ or } P = \frac{E}{D + A + K}$$

P = probability
E = event
D = data
C = conditions
K = knowledge
A = assumptions

The $P(E|D,A,K)$ could be interpreted as a presumable rational where the likelihood of an event is discussed. This is an important facet for clinical research, especially where probability could be used to report the likelihood of a diagnosis or treatment outcome. Probabilistic diagnosis is more commonly used in communicable disease research where selective populations are randomly selected to evaluate the presence or absence of a virus. In this type of scenario, the data tend to be laboratory samples. A useful example is cited below:

A population has 0.2% of their people infected by a virus. The laboratory tests indicate a positive yield of 98% of infected people and 1% in noninfected. The tests would be carried out on random people within the population.

This would imply the following:
Step 1

$$P = \frac{Ip}{Vp}$$

P = Probability
Ip = Positive laboratory result
Vp = A carrier of the virus
K = Knowledge
A = Assumption
Step 2

$$P = \frac{Ip}{Vp}$$

$P = 0.98$ and $P = 0.01$.

If the test indicates a positive result, there is an interest to assess the probability of the individual being a carrier of the virus. To assess this probability, the positive result, assumption, and knowledge of the prevalence of the virus within the said population are required. This would mean:

Step 3

$$P = \frac{Vp}{K} = 0.002$$

This could be transformed to probability algebra which is associated with the Bayes theorem to demonstrate yield.

Model

A typical example of the Bayes theorem is as follows:

$P(\text{Infected}|\text{positive})$

$$= \frac{P(\text{Infected}|\text{positive})P(\text{Infected})}{P(P|\text{Infected})P(\text{Infected}) + P(P|\text{Infected})P(\text{Infected})}$$

$$P = \frac{Vp}{Ip + A + K} = 0.164$$

In other words, the probabilities described have conditional measures of uncertainty therefore, the interpretation remains the same. Hence, the final model can be used to evaluate uncertainty with a person testing positive is in fact infected, and by definition the proportion of those infected in the population to be 16.4%. This means the probability reported can be validated further with a diagnosis step by way of completing a test to show a positive result.

Prediction

Prediction is an important component in clinical medicine. Therefore, using prediction models to assess probability is a vital component in clinical research. Both epidemiological and clinical trial data could be used to carry-forth predictions. An example is demonstrated below:

$R =$ Count
$E =$ Event
$N =$ Number of replications
$D =$ Data
$J =$ Replication
$A =$ Assumptions
$K =$ Knowledge

In the event of an experiment, events (E) could take place a number of times (R). These could be replicated (J) in numerous

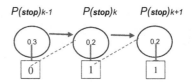

Fig. 3.4 A prediction model based on assumptions and knowledge.

situations (N), forecasting the number of counts by which the event could take place. Predictions on discrete quantity based on existing data, formulated assumptions (A) on mechanistic probability would provide the number of times the event would take place along with relevant knowledge (K). An example of this shown in Fig. 3.4.

Clinical versus statistical significance

Clinical research studies often report clinical and statistical significance in different ways. Most clinical research publications report efficacy, effectiveness, or efficiency. Within the context of statistical versus clinical significance, these could have differing meanings. Efficacy assesses the intervention being explored such as the drug, medical device, and/or programme using a two-arm clinical trial. Effectiveness evaluates the intervention being explored within the context of the population primarily using a clinical trial. Efficiency assesses the cost-effectiveness and reports on the socio-economic value of the intervention. The key to reporting these accurately is not just about the use of appropriate statistical tests, but the clinical questions and the eligibility criteria used to gather the data. To achieve accurate efficacy, efficiency, and effectiveness reporting, understanding the measures of central tendency and dispersion is important.

The presence of harmonisation between statistical and clinical significance is commonly observed in well-designed research. Statistical significance represents reliability of the study findings which could demonstrate the impact on clinical practice. There are pitfalls when there is a lack of differentiation between the statistical and clinical significance and are a common issue in publications. Measures of statistical significance include P values and confidence intervals where the probability of the study findings shows the magnitude of the effect. Clinical significance on the other hand is interpreted on the practical significance of the quantifiable effects reported by way of the statistical analysis. A casing point to remember is that statistical significance should

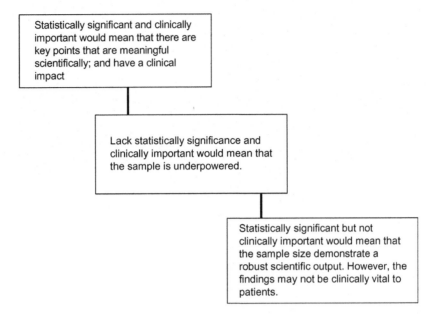

Fig. 3.5 A scenario tree related to statistical significance.

be prioritised in clinical research especially when reporting effect size. For example, even within large data sets, a small difference within the statistical analyses could become a significant finding clinically. A good example of this would be within rare-disease-based research. A scenario tree is in Fig. 3.5 (Table 3.2).

All researchers should have at least a working understanding of algebra to enable statistical inference issues to be resolved at the design and analysis stage. Deviations of assumptions are avoidable by way of using a statistical analysis map. The misinterpretation of statistical conclusions does not require mastery of advanced mathematics although the use of these from a practical concept perspective is useful when discussing study findings and their generalisability within populations.

Monte Carlo simulation

The Monte Carlo methods are considered a computational technique despite the fact that their inception is associated with mathematical constructs in which the solutions are mathematically provided using random samples. This method was born out of Physicists in the 1940s, where it was used to solve particle transport problems and was considered as a revolutionary step to

Table 3.2 Clinical versus statistical significance.

Statistical tests	Application	Statistical significance	Clinical significance	Considerations
Effect size	Demonstrates a meaningful relationship between different groups or variables	P-Values and confidence intervals based on the observations identified within the study sample	Measure observed based on the correlation of two variables such as mean difference or probability	For example, a significant effect size could mean a significant practical significance of the outcome and generalisability. If the effect size is insignificant, the findings could have limitations
Clarity of the data analysis	A high-quality data analysis should have a robust method and methodology	Objective	Subjective	The data analysis should be aligned to the scope of the research question. Synthesising the evidence based on the methods and methodology is vital to show reasonable conclusions. Homogeneity or heterogeneity of the data analysis should be discussed, and where possible a further analysis such as a sensitivity analysis completed
Risk of bias	Risk of bias should be used in studies with or without a comparison. Risk of bias should be used to ensure methodological rigour and reliability of the findings	Biases can be identified and assessed within the samples. A sensitivity analysis should further assist with managing any biases	Biases could be explained as often clinical outcomes can be defined medically using many parameters	Reducing subjectivity and ensuring the study outputs remain objective is important. Fata should be verified independently prior to the data analysis. Any risk of bias should be assessed using validated risk of bias tool
Null hypothesis	Null hypothesis is a conjuncture to assess two phenomena. Its' primary application would be to assess plausibility of a hypothesis used in a research study	Assumption the lack of a statistical significance which is likely to be due to the absence of a relationship observed with the data set	A nullified hypothesis means the lack of clinical significance within the dataset	For example, this is an important aspect to evaluate with public health research to assess the strength of the evidence

Table 3.2 Clinical versus statistical significance—cont'd

Statistical tests	Application	Statistical significance	Clinical significance	Considerations
P-Value		Probability within the sample size used for the analysis. For example, if the P value is 0.040, there is 4.0% chance the observed difference within the sample size	Results can be statistically significant but still minimal from a clinical perspective. Therefore, it is important to interpret the statistically significant or insignificant P-values in the practical sense. The P-value on its own should not be used to demonstrate clinical significance	For example, systematic reviews reporting effect size is vital to consider before conclusions around statistical and clinical significance is made
Sample size	Sample size is vital for all research conducted, and its relationship with the findings. Small sample sizes can be challenging to justify as the scientific relevance and generalisability to a wider population can be limited. Using sample size as a key application tool in research is important	The larger the sample size, the likelihood of the results reflecting randomness and generalisability of the findings would be significant	The generalisability of the statistical findings and their relevance from a clinical perspective that could increase validity and reliability	This is an important facet of conducting a scientifically and clinically justifiable research study
Confidence intervals	Confidence intervals are used in a variety of research studies to determine the accuracy of the estimated statistics	This is a frequentist statistics method	Confidence intervals along with P-values could provide a range of possible effects that could demonstrate the relevance of the findings to patients	For example, 95% Confidence interval for a probability of a mean value suggests that a population mean can be between 9 and 11. High level of confidence would indicate a narrower interval

Continued

Table 3.2 Clinical versus statistical significance—cont'd

Statistical tests	Application	Statistical significance	Clinical significance	Considerations
Reliability change index	This is a psychometric criterion that is a concept measure and assessment	This statistical measure used to assess a change over a specific time period		Primarily within clinical trials and prospective clinical research studies could benefit from the use of this method
Selective reporting	Selective reporting introduces biases and unreliable results in a research study. This is an application that should be avoided	Selective reporting can be a problem due to a number of factors including a rigid inclusion/exclusion criterion as well as multiple testing when the dataset is minimal	Selective reporting reports to minimal clinical impact. Any 'cherry-picking' when reporting findings also lead to incorrect interpretation of the hypothesis and relevance of the dataset to the disease and population being studies	For example, ensuring systematic approaches with accurate eligibility criteria when finalising the sample size would be useful. The PICO approach could also assist with avoiding selective reporting
Odds ratio (OR) also referred to as prevalence ratio	Compares prevalence based on exposures as described by the outcome. Therefore, this is a measure of association	OR is a statistical measure of association between an exposure and outcomes	ORs demonstrate the odds of an outcome in a study due to a specific exposure in comparison to the outcome when the same exposure is absent. This relationship is clinically quantifiable to report the strength of the association	Misused when comparing incidence where exposures are categorised. ORs become invalid if independent assumptions are violated
Relative risk (*RR*) also referred to hazard ratio, incidence ratio or risk ratio	Compare the incidence of diseases based on the exposure. Therefore, this is a measure of association	RR or risk ratio is a statistical measure of a risk that occurred in one group in comparison to another. If RR is insignificant than 1, there is a negative association where the exposure may be	Using RR with odds ratios is more useful clinically to report risk measures that are associated between outcomes and exposures	Misused when comparing prevalence when datasets are categorised based on outcomes. RR is invalid in the presence of violated independent assumptions

Table 3.2 Clinical versus statistical significance—cont'd

Statistical tests	Application	Statistical significance	Clinical significance	Considerations
		acting as a protective factor. If RR is equal to 1, the exposure may lack any effect on risk. This would mean a lack of association between the exposure and the outcome		
Attributable risk (AR) also referred to as excess risk or attributable portion	Quantify the difference between incidence rates across multiple exposures. Therefore, this is a measure of association	AR is a simple statistical calculation which can be subtracted from risk of the nonexposed group and the exposed group	Commonly reported in epidemiological research and clinically useful to report risk differences in a population. Mortality or incidence due to a particular disease can be reported using AR. An insignificant	AR should be used primarily in incidence studies where the exposures in the control group would be deemed a normal exposure. AR would be invalid in the presence of violated independent assumptions
Person Chi-square test	Independence test used to compare the proportional distribution of outcome variables between groups based on a predictor variable	This is a statistical test used with categorical data to report the observed difference and the data arose by chance	This test can be used to report observed distributions as a result of chance. Clinically, this is useful to report the presence or absence of any symptoms associated with a disease	This method should not be used for paired data but useful for incidence or prevalence studies. Invalid in the presence of violated independent assumptions
Kappa statistic	Reliability test to report proportion of agreement in paired data	Interrater reliability is tested using the Kappa statistic method. The statistical importance of this data is associated with the reliability of the data gathered for a study where the variables measured are accurate	Clinical interpretation of a Kappa statistic is useful in the context of comparing radiology scans, workforce research and diagnostic variability amongst multiple clinicians	This test can be developed for paired data where an independence is absent

Continued

Table 3.2 Clinical versus statistical significance—cont'd

Statistical tests	Application	Statistical significance	Clinical significance	Considerations
McNemar's Chi square test	Proportional disagreement test used to assess disagreements in case-matched or repeated measures	Demonstrates the difference between correlated aspects in a study		Suitable for datasets where there is a repeated measure or case matching in the presence of a hypothesis of proportions between discordant factors
Combined quality improvement ratio	Improvement test that could be used to improve worsening pairs at random			This is specific to paired data based on repeated measures or case matching
Analysis of variance (ANOVA)	Equality of means test between groups or measures at specific time points. This meant means of continuous variables could be compared	This can be completed with repeated measures		ANOVA is highly sensitive to unusually distributed data

generate pseudo random numbers to conduct an experimental analysis than a physical experiment. The realisation of the use of this method in clinical research was often considered in complex clinical areas due to difficulties in recruiting patients and retaining them for the period of a study. It was further understood that the applicability of the method could also solve epidemiological issues where there was a paucity of high-quality data and the missing data issues threatened meaningful probabilistic outputs to be demonstrated. The Monte Carlo simulation is a mathematical method where multiplicity of probability is estimated to report possible outcomes on uncertain events. The Monte Carlo simulation method is becoming more useful in clinical research where statistical inference could be encoded posterior probability distribution. The Monte Carlo simulation methods are a general group of computational techniques for mathematical problems by way of random sampling. This method can be used to synthesise quantitative data for clinical trials and epidemiology studies.

The physics community continues to advance the Monte Carlo methodology, especially by way of the Markov Chain Monte Carlo (MCMC) where the use of discrete time to generate dependent variables could allow integration with experimental data to optimise the evaluation of high-dimensional integrals. The Monte Carlo method also generates complex probability distributions which can be useful to predict disease outcomes for both communicable and noncommunicable diseases. The theoretical and methodology development of this application has led to its use in Bayesian statistics, more specifically with the inferential technique where normalisation of constants in samples can be considered through proposal distribution. Within some disease areas where complex symptomatology is apparent, designing normalised data sets could be a challenge. The MCMC could provide a solution to this high-dimensional integral issue. A Bayesian model can show an unknown parameter using distribution rather than a fixed estimate of time. The parameters of the model have distributions and remain probabilistic such as parameters associated with coefficients linked to covariates within a regression model.

Data models are becoming more complex as a result of the changing landscape in clinical research. Therefore, statistical inference is becoming a common issue that influences researchers to use novel methods due to limitations noted in traditional techniques. There are two primary classes of statistical problems of integration and optimisation, where characterising distributions that aid the calculation of outcomes becomes the fundamental usefulness in Epidemiology and Clinical trial data. Within the Bayesian paradigm, the Monte Carlo method is a common technique. This can be completed using four key steps:

Step 1: identify the transfer equation
A quantitative model is required to model the activity, plan, or process that is explored by way of a mathematical expression. This is referred to as the transfer equation or a model created for a designed experiment or regression analysis. The equations developed can have multiple responses that are dependent on one another in cases where there are multiple outcomes or exposures reported.

Step 2: input parameters should be defined
The transfer equation could determine the distribution of the data. The data inputs may show binomial, uniformal, or triangular distribution. The distribution parameters for inputs should be determined individually.

Step 3: develop the simulation
For a true simulation, a large and random data set should be created, for example, with a sample size of 100,000. The random data points would simulate values over a period of time for each input leading to the development of the mathematical model.

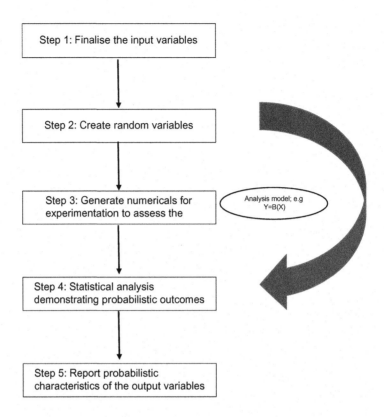

Fig. 3.6 The Monte Carlo method.

Step 4: analyse the process outputs

The simulated data should be explored with the transfer equation to report the outcomes. A reliable indication of the output would be demonstrated through the model developed.

The schematic representation of the steps is demonstrated in Fig. 3.6.

3.3 Epidemiology statistics

The science of Epidemiology began with analytical tools and statistical methods to oversee health and disease profiles across multiple populations. In the early 19th century, Epidemiology developed over five phases that overlapped with one another, as demonstrated in Fig. 3.7.

The pioneers of Epidemiology are considered to be Frenchman Louis Rene Villerme (1782–1863) and Englishman William Farr (1807–83). Farr was appointed as the compiler of abstracts to

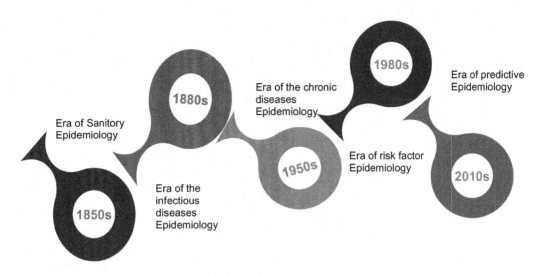

Fig. 3.7 The timeline over which epidemiology developed.

the Registrar General to develop medical statistics which would enhance preventative medicine within England. He analysed large mortality data sets comparing various diseases in different geographical locations. This work led to demonstrating the socio-economical and disease phenomenon, especially during urbanisation in Great Britain. Farr and Villerme both reflected libertarian ideology where moral habits of all social classes were important in the implementation of preventative disease interventions with laws and regulations. However, these views contrasted that of those in The Epidemiological Society of London. The influence of the European revolution prompted political, social, and economic justice which influenced the remedial action for water supply, sanitation, and control of food, hygiene, and healthy working environments. Hence, the 1850s are referred to as the *Era of Sanitary Statistics* that was based on the *miasmatic theory* of disease, also referred to as the *cause-and-effect* paradigm.

British epidemiology studies grew more robust by the early 20th century by way of both observation and deductive methods. The changes over a period of time, social disparities, morbidity, mortality, and regional differences were important, especially part of the microbiological revolution with advancement of pathophysiology giving rise to the germ theory. As a result, this is referred to as the *Era of the Infectious Diseases* that led to further research in identifying microorganisms responsible for contagious diseases and their study in laboratory environments.

Kristian Feyer Andvord (1855–1934) was influenced by ideas from 40 years before tuberculosis (TB) spread due to concerns about geographical variations among birth cohorts across time. This was conceptualised as '*generation studies*' by Andvord, leading to the introduction of *cohort analysis*. This cohort analysis became a key epidemiological analytical tool since the 1940s. Andvord aimed to find out the pattern of infection transmission and the manifestation into a disease. He also determined TB transmission by age instead of gender or vocation which led to the formulation of '*the TB Act of 1900*'.

Decades have added to the advancement of Epidemiology by way of using sophisticated mathematical-statistical and biometrics methods. Mathematical methods to evaluate biological patterns, evolution, genetic processes, and variation prepared a *Mecca of learning* for better integration of medical statistics into integrated medicine. This led to the interest to the *Era of Chronic Diseases epidemiology*. Austin Bradford Hill (1897–1991), a statistician, and Richard Doll (1912–2005), a physician, conducted the first smoking and lung cancer epidemiology study promoting objective statistical methods leading to long-term assessment of cancer outcomes.

The 21st century has given rise to the Era of Risk Factor Epidemiology which is a highly specialised area that uses mathematical methods and statistical analyses moving away from more conventional methods.

Descriptive statistics

Ecological studies tend to employ a descriptive approach to analyse a data series report measures of characteristics of the population and disease being explored using variables such as medication. Correlation coefficients such as Pearson's 'r', Spearman's 'T', or Kendall's 'K' are commonly used to report linear relationships between the exposure or predictor and the disease or outcomes. The value of these can vary between positive 1 and negative 1. The positive 1 demonstrates an effective correlation where the exposure or predictor increases with the disease or outcomes. The negative 1 shows an inverse correlation where the predictor or exposure increases and the outcome decreases. Case reports and case series commonly rely on descriptive statistics where percentile, mean, median, mode, standard deviation, kurtosis, variance, and range are reported. This is often referred to as conventional statistics and is also used in sociology, political science, and engineering in addition to medicine.

Cause-and-effect paradigm

Causation is a vital concept in epidemiology. Despite a variety of discussions, a standard and unified concept remains to be seen. The presence of multiple definitions could be due to the variability in the context of scientific and clinical practices as the underlying concept of causation could be different.

A probabilistic definition of causation is an alternative to determinism for establishing necessary and sufficient causation. Probabilistic causation could explain indeterministic processes which provide a theoretical basis to construct models of interaction. In the context of drugs, this could be in relation to dose–response in terms of quantitative values in a continuum format. The probability of the effect could be described mathematically, therefore more suited to report effect measurement. Counterfactuals are another facet of component cause or probabilistic definition. Advocacy for counterfactual definitions of causation includes contrasts demonstrated between one outcome due to one condition and a second outcome as a result of another condition. To articulate this further, distinction between correlation and causation is made. Thus, there could be confusion between ontology and epistemology which impacts the distinction between intervention and the subsequent relative observations as well as the frequency of these. In addition, scientific inference could be considered as a causal model associated with a specific phenomenon which could assist with generalising outcomes.

Mendelian randomisation

Mendelian randomisation is an epidemiological method that can measure variation in genes to assess causal effects of modifiable exposures of a disease. Thus, this is a useful method to explore causation and correlation to understand disease mechanisms. This is a reliable method of analysis when applied to a valid genetic sample comprising instrumental variables to evaluate if a risk factor can have a causal effect on an observed outcome [23,24]. This statistical methodology uses genetic variants as proxy measures for clinical interventions. The variants are used analogously to random assignment as demonstrated in Fig. 3.8.

Mendalian randomisation is minimally affected by confounding or reverse causation in comparison to other observational

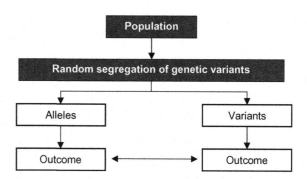

Fig. 3.8 How genetic variants are assigned via Mendelian randomisation.

studies. This approach uses assumptions; thus, further methods are required to address the plausibility of these within the context of the results being applied to clinical practice. Thus, combining these with an evidence synthesis approach along with a sensitivity analysis could strengthen any conclusions and clinical

Table 3.3 A glossary of concepts and common terms used when reporting Mendelian randomised studies.

	Concept	Description
1	Instrumental variables	These are variables linked to the risk factors of interest within a study. These are unrelated to confounders yet impact the outcome byway of the risk factor. Instrument variables could be any disease trait and isn't specific to genetic variants [25]
2	Mendelian randomisation	This is a technique where genetic variants are used as instrumental variables to assess effects of modifiable risks for a disease [26]
3	Instruments	This implies the use of more than 1 genetic variant within the analysis
4	Instrument bias	This incurs when the analysis includes one or more variants within a proportion of a sample size [27]
5	Pleiotropic effects	These are effects observed in multiple biological pathways where it affects the outcome by way of another trail (indirect) or the pathway being explored (direct). This is known as horizontal pleiotropy. The indirect affect is referred to as vertical pleiotropy [28]. Horizontal pleiotropic effects are a violation of instrumental variable assumptions as the effects of the genetic variants are nonexclusive. Vertical pleiotropy on the other hand Is not an issue for mendelian randomisation studies as a single factor influences a downstream outcome [27,28]
6	Allele scores	These are the scores linked to all the alleles associated with risk factors being explored. The variants identified are usually within large sample sizes and the statistical power could be increased by way of weighting variants [29,30]

recommendations. Key concepts and a glossary of terminologies used in the context of Mendelian randomised studies are indicated in Table 3.3.

There are key statistical methods that can be considered when designing a Mendelian randomisation study, and these are as follows [26]:

- Single sample mendelian randomisation uses a single data set within the instrumental variable analysis to report causal estimates of the risk factor associated with the relevant outcome.
- Two-sample Mendelian randomisation uses two different data sets to estimate instrument-risk factors and instrument-outcome associated to report causal effects. This method significantly increases the statistical power by including multiple data sets.
- Mendelian randomisation Egger regression reports the pleiotropic effects independent of the genetic variant effects on risk factors of interest.
- Genetic instruments used have multiple properties where testing between the observation and Mendelian randomisation estimate is reported. Hausman test is used for continuous outcomes in a single Mendelian randomisation.
- Instrument strength is assessed using tests to explore the association between the risk factor and instrument. Partial F statistic and R^2 are reported as part of this test.

Instrument validation is key within the Mendelian studies which are important and based on three assumptions:

- Relevance assumption: This describes the risk fact association with genetic variants. In the case of a single sample Mendelian study, risk difference or r^2 and partial F statistic could be used as a tool to report plausibility [31,32]. For two-sample Mendalian studies, variants associated with risk factors would be useful tools to evaluate plausibility [33].
- Independence assumption [32].
- Exclusion restriction.

Spatial statistics

Spatial statistics is an extension of descriptive statistics where it is commonly applied to geographical or preclinical data. In the 1970s, Tobler's law was used to describe the first laws of geography which described **'everything is related to everything else but near things are more related than distant things'**. This concept led to the development of spatial statistics. Spatial statistics is commonly used in medical physics which is useful in the development and testing of radiological equipment, such as scanners

[22]. In addition, this can be used as a statistical modelling and prediction method to report spatial interaction or as part of a pattern analysis. Thus, this method can be used within epidemiological studies and clinical trials [34]. For example, cluster randomised trials use geographical regions as a unit of randomisation although explicit spatial distribution of observation is rarely reported and can be important to report spillover or herd effects for communicable diseases. Unreported spillover effects could increase biases and thereby reduce the quality of the trial findings [9]. Spatial effect in this context is valuable as it demonstrates locational variation between the phenomena of interest. This could further assist with reporting treatment effect estimations within a specific location. Global spatial effect estimates are uncertain as it could be underestimated or overestimated. The debate around spatial effects impacted the early predictions made about herd immunity during the COVID-19 pandemic due to spatial dependence. Spatial dependence is a key concept where a single variable could be related to another close value within the same variable set. Spatial effects can be analysed using spatial variables and models, as described below:

- Spatial variables: Straight line distance and density are two types of spatial variables that describe temporal dimensions. Denotation of space as a variable can be used in a differential equation, as follows:

$$D = \gamma d + \varepsilon$$

γ = effect of change in variable D.
D was defined as either a straight line distance or density.

  - Straight line distance is an estimated spatial effect reported by way of measuring the distance between a location and participants [35,36]. Locations could sometimes be a characteristic that may affect an outcome or a participant. For example, within a clinical trial context, the distance between a control and interventional participant could be used to report the discordant observation [36]. In addition, distances could also be categorised to calculate standardise morbidity or mortality rate.
  - Density [37] is a measure of the effect of density surrounding the participants. Factors associated with density could impact the outcomes such as counts or proportion over a period of time. This method could be applied to focus on treatment density or risk of infection. For example, intervention density could be measured based on the number of households as demonstrated by Lenhart and colleagues.

On the other hand, Miguel and colleagues [38] measured treatment density within a 6 km radius of a school in addition to reporting counts as part of their primary analysis. Ali and colleagues [39] reported a count density and proportion as part of their typhoid prevalence and private practitioners within a specific neighbourhood. Chao and colleagues [40] developed and tested a new method to report spatial effects in cluster randomised trials referred to as '**potential exposure**'. Potential exposure refers to the sum of relative risks and controls spatial variation. In the context of Chao and colleagues' study, potential exposure was reported for people that lived within 100 m of one another as well as its use to report heterogeneous risk factors within the trial.

- Spatial models: this is a method representing the underlying spatial process [41]. Spatial process could be measured and effectively estimated. Spatial models can be structured with random effect. Random effect within negative binomial models is useful to report spatial patterns as demonstrated by Alexander and colleagues and Fig. 3.9 where the spatial structure was shown as a matrix that included the observations that were connected to one another [42]. A distance decaying parameter within the covariance structure in the random effect was used to report the estimated half-distance. Half-distance is where spatial correlation halves. Spatial effects impact the precision and value of estimated intervention effects although spatial models could also fit better than a standard cluster randomised effect model, as demonstrated by Chao and colleagues. Spatial effects may need to be adjusted and could be used in a variety of disease areas although communicable diseases appear to be the most befitting for this type of methodology use.

	A	B	C	D
A	0	3	1	8
B	3	0	1	4
C	1	1	0	6
D	8	4	6	0

$Y = X\gamma + U + e$ *where* Y is vector of the outcome.
X is the design matrix
e represents error terms
γ is a vector of coefficients
U represents a random effect

Where $U \sim MVN\ (0, \theta^2_u \Sigma)$

$\Sigma_{ij} = e^{-d_{ij}/\theta}$ where d_{ij} that shows the distance between observations *j* and *i* and θ as a scale parameter.

Fig. 3.9 A spatial model based on four clinical trials.

Table 3.4 Examples of spatial epidemiology.

Data	Description
Field of epidemiology	Surveys around disease occurrence gathered via digital sensors including GPS
Big-data	Data gathered within databases from a variety of sources including routinely gathered clinical data and/or research repository data
Clinical disease	Registries, health surveys, surveillance, and data depositories
Demographics	Socio-demographic and socio-economic
Environmental	Data surrounding air and/or water quality, climate, and geology

Spatial epidemiology

Spatial epidemiology is a subcategory that quantifies and aims to explain geographical variation observed in diseases and their association with socio-economic, genetic, demographic, behavioural, and environmental factors. Disease mapping is a key feature and method used in spatial epidemiology where this predicts disease outcome patterns across a single or multiple geographical areas including those that could stratified by risk. The same methods could be used to explore the understanding of disease causation. Table 3.4 indicates example of spatial epidemiology studies and the data utilised.

Spatial correlation

Inferential issues associated with spatial data are a common problem leading to data quality issues. Spatial correlation demonstrates identical measures from varying locations, thus confirmation of the presence would violate independent and identical distribution of the data. Thus, conclusions where spatial correlation is present would be false. Thus, statistical techniques need to be carefully sought to ensure the validity of the results in the presence of spatial correlation.

GIS and other statistical packages could conduct area-level data analysis including Moran's I, Geary's C, Tango's Maximised Excess Events Test (MEET), spatial scan statistics, and localised indicators of spatial association (LISA) [43,44].

Moran's I in particular [43] could assess global clustering which could be defined as follows:

$$\text{Moran's} = \frac{1}{\sum_{i=1}^{I}(z_i - \bar{z})^2} \times \frac{\sum_{i=1}^{I}\sum_{j=1}^{I}w_{ij}(z_i - \bar{z})(z_j - \bar{z})}{\sum_{i=1}^{I}\sum_{j=1}^{I}w_{ij}}$$

Z_i would be considered as an observation value at each area $i=1$, whilst I areas, z remains as the mean value. I represents the number of areas, and w_{ij} indicates the statistical weights associated with adjacent localities [45,46]. Values of Moran's I range between -1 (dispersed) and $+1$ (clustering) where values at 0 lack spatial correlation [43].

Geary's C is another similar spatial correlation method that is defined as below:

$$\text{Geary's C} = \frac{I - 1}{\sum_{i=1}^{I}(z_i - \bar{z})^2} \times \frac{\sum_{i=1}^{I}\sum_{j=1}^{I}w_{ij}(z_i - z_j)^2}{2\sum_{i=1}^{I}\sum_{j=1}^{I}w_{ij}}$$

Geary's C ranges between 0 and 2 where 1 means there would be a lack of spatial correlation. Values <1 demonstrate the presence of spatial correlation whilst >1 shows the lack of it [44].

Tango's MEET uses the excess event test (EET) based on an excess of events (observed minus expected) where higher weights are proximal and o_i and p_i observed count and population [46]. O_{TOT} and P_{TOT} represent the count and population where d_{ij} demonstrates the distance between two areas of i and j [47,48]. However, λ could influence outcomes where significant values demonstrate sensitivity to determine large geographical clusters, and vice versa.

$$\text{EET} = \sum_{i}\sum_{j}e^{-\frac{4d_{ij}^2}{\lambda^2}}\left(o_i - \frac{p_i o_{TOT}}{P_{TOT}}\right)\left(o_j - \frac{p_j o_{TOT}}{P_{TOT}}\right)$$

The equation for LISA is as follows:

$$I_i = (z_i - \bar{z}) \times \sum_{j \in J_i}^{n} w_{ij}(z_i - \bar{z})^2$$

LISA have multiple versions using common global indicators that are shared with Geary's C. This method is useful to indicate the scope of remarkable spatial clustering within the area of interest. The sum of LISA produces proportionate global statistics. However, there are disadvantages of using this method in relation to multiple testing given an individual statistical test is required for each region included in a sample. Small regions and rates could remain unstable at the peril of spurious significance. These issues could be resolved with a Bonferroni adjustment where correlations between LISA can become conservative.

Global clustering methods could be used to be associated within the regions of choice indicating an overall pattern to the outcomes [46]. In comparison, clustering methods could detect locations that are statistically significant within a spatial cluster indicating risk of disease.

Neighbourhood

Spatial correlation could be discussed by way of describing a neighbourhood using a model composed of different areas including any internal and external influences recorded on observations [49,50]. Defining an area within a *neighbourhood* was based on spatial adjacency by way of using the shortest distance between two points [51]. A weighted mechanism can be used to demonstrate the impact of the neighbours reported as an estimate for the area being explored [52,53]. For example, zero indicates no weight relationship whilst above zero means two adjacent areas could be neighbours [54]. The weights can be placed in a matrix that includes dimensions for the areas being explored. Similarity of regions could be calculated using a diagonal that is set at zero [55]. Thus, neighbourhood structures could exert influence on spatial analyses.

Unsmoothed estimates

Unsmoothed estimates are the *raw* estimates that can be calculated for small areas. Generated values can be displayed as counts using a dotted map within the area of interest [56]. Mapping the counts remains insufficient to understand disease risk unless population size and structure can be adjusted by reporting rates as a reflection of risk [57]. There are different types of rates explored although crude rates, proportions, and percentages are commonly reported. Crude rates can be calculated as follows:

$$CR_i = \frac{O_i}{P_i}$$

where ith area ($i = 1, \ldots.I$), O_i represents the observed counts within, and P_i indicates the number of people. Small crude rates are reported as per constant.

An alternative method would be to report rates within an adjusted population structure where variables such as age are standardised based on the counts of disease or the expected counts based on a standard population. These can be further adjusted to variables specific to the area being explored such as socioeconomic status and age. Direct standardisation may focus on estimating the number of deaths observed within the standard population when rates of disease within a specific age group are reported by way of weighting the sex and age-specific rates for an area with a structured population [58]. On the other hand, indirect standardisation uses estimated mortality on the basis of the study population contracting the disease at a similar rate. Thus, indirect rate increases the stratified population per area explored by the known disease rates based on an existing population. This evaluation process leads to standardised morbidity or mortality ratio (SMR). This equation was demonstrated by

$$SMR_i = \frac{O_i}{E_i}$$

where ith are $i = 1, ... I$, O_i indicates observed counts within a specific area (i) with an overall disease rate based on an age-specific population of P of area i and summarising m age groups (where *M being the maximum age groups)* and excluding sex [36–58]. Observed disease counts are represented by O_{refm} and P_{refm} indicates the control population age group as m. The evaluation equation is as follows:

$$E_i = \sum^{m=1} \frac{O_{refm} \times P_m}{P_{refm}}$$

3.4 Disease mapping methods

Disease mapping is defined as a group of methods to report small area estimations using spatial settings alongside the assumed positive spatial correlations between observations to report disease spread [59]. This is primarily a data visualisation method when showing geographical distribution. In essence, borrowed information from neighbours is used to develop geographic information systems (GISs) and epidemiological models. These are commonly used to report patterns of disease such as the instance of outbreaks of communicable disease [52,59]. Thus, disease mapping methods are important to report incidence and prevalence to promote public health and are a common method to promote population sciences. The following are key disease mapping methods in use:

- Clustering
- Ecological
- Risk

Clustering

One of the first examples of disease mapping was John Snow's studies of the London Cholera epidemic from 1854 where a cluster of cases were shown around Broad Street. During this time, aetiology and epidemiology of cholera were unknown as the isolation of the Cholera bacterium preceded by 45 years. Meticulous attention to clinical details and environmental factors allowed John Snow to demonstrate that the spread of Cholera was due to contaminated water from the river Thames. However, cluster detection can be complicated for some diseases. There are several methods that can be used to address two specific problems of cluster detection of the presence or absence of clusters and spatial location as well as the extent of these. However, clustering methods can be primarily categorised as General clustering and Focused clustering. General clustering methods test hypothesis to report clusters based on general tendencies in data observed whilst focused clustering test hypothesis using prespecified spatial locations. Both categories use spatial methods demonstrated the use of case-event models and subsequent data analysis can be useful to understand disease transmission although this may be subjected to ecological bias.

Spatial cluster modelling is a useful approach that Lawson et al. discuss to demonstrate focused clustering when mapping a disease. Whilst there are various general clustering methods, it is vital to test the hypothesis of the data distribution's tendency. However, spatial cluster detection when monitored, incidence could be higher than anticipated especially for cases such as influenza [60]. Part of the reasoning for this could be the underreporting of flu cases in healthcare records as not every patient would be required to be seen by a physician. However, there are spatial cluster detection methods that are disease-independent. A common use of this can be through syndromic data which are commonly used in respiratory syndromes observed by way of hospital admissions or the sale of over-the-counter medication from pharmacies. This can be a useful way to predict outbreaks as well by way of a population-based approach such as *an-at-risk* population specific to a geographical region that can be adjusted to covariate effects such as age, gender, and biological sex [60]. Another approach would be *expectation-based* which uses estimated case numbers within a specific geographical location by way of a model developed by past data. Wagner and colleagues discussed this approach where the estimate could be much larger than the actuals. An important difference between the *at-risk* and *expectation-based* would be the applicability of these to understand global epidemics or pandemics. In some instances, a combination of the two could be useful for healthcare providers and policy-makers to allocate resources and stock up any required medications [60].

Resolution of data presented in a disease map can be useful to understand regional differences. This type of method can be used to report census enumeration data and was popularised further in COVID-19 pandemic transmission. There are possible incompatibilities that could impact the findings including location ambiguity. Geographical analysis conducted should report *P*-values to indicate overall clustering. Other approaches include the use of disease aetiology to analyse the data or with approximations using the Monte Carlo simulation method which can support extensive power calculation to generate more meaningful outputs.

P-Values can be generated using a number of tests although there is much debate around the validity of these approaches especially when demonstrating clustering in cancers. A good example is the Moran's test or the conventional Gaussian approximation or simple randomisation analysis used when reporting rates of incidence or raking tends to be factually incorrect even in instances where risk is considered as a constant. In such instances, the Monte Carlo versions on multivariate hypergeometric distributions would be better equipped to report geographical incidence rates [60]. The disadvantage with this approach is that it is computationally intensive where the sample population is significant and thereby intensive in terms of resource use.

Ecological

Ecological approaches can be used with hierarchical Bayesian modelling and spatial interaction modelling with covariates assessed with or without errors. Bayesian models are more realistic and outcomes are more structured in nature which could include cause/effects. However, model validation requires sensitivity analysis to ensure the reliability of the model without any overparametrisation where covariates may be considered as confounders. The risk of overadjustment in these instances is another aspect that needs to be carefully addressed by using methods such as spatial smoothing and estimating interactions with spatial parameters. There could be multiple rationales that could be used to assess model features such as:

- Selected model should comprise measured covariates where the posterior is checked using spatial part. If the results are positive, model phenomena would be accurate for the study

- A regression model can have a spatial part which lacks an explanation in the presence of covariates. In this instance, spatial features may be associated with covariates that are neither defined nor measured. Epidemiologically, such a model where spatial residual is present cannot be explained although there would be a clinical justification available. Thus, retaining a spatial part in such a model can seem cautious and conclusions suboptimal.
- Strong spatially structured effects can be a key characteristic of data gathered in a study. For example, vicinity can be an interpretive factor in infectious disease studies. This type of spatial model can be transferrable in the use of other diseases, where the informative nature could further assess hypotheses such as the presence or absence of an infectious disease within childhood cancers.

Inferential ideas with two models can also be introduced when using ecological methods where data could be managed using novel methods by way of grids and scales circumventing aggregation of information that has minimal scales. Another new approach could be to use nonparametric inferences in spatial auto models. These models have covariates that harmonise spatial interactions. This is commonly evaluated using computational software.

Misinterpretation of disease maps is another issue when using ecological methods in particular where these lack clarity on underlying assumptions and models. Public health organisations and policy-makers should consider all approaches carefully to ensure the relevance of the findings to the populations.

Risk

Case–control studies commonly use risk analysis. Poisson assumption is a common method that can be used on count data report area-specific rates. Poisson, also referred to as a binomial random variable based linear model, could be used with a log or logit link function. In this model, geographically specific covariates (x_i) can be used with any associated parameters (β). Counts of the disease (Y_i) within the model are set for a specific geographical location $i = 1, ..., I$ with a partitioning domain D. The model also includes people at risk (n_i) or the expected cases at risk that may have a disease transmission null model (E_i). For example, circular annuli can be used to determine the lung cancer risk in a region with high pollution. This can be furthered in a multivariate analysis which could include information on participant's occupation and smoking. Ecological fallacy should be considered when discussing the results in the analysis. The Poisson model using fixed effects could be used as follows [61]:

$$Y_i | \zeta_i \overset{ind}{\sim} \text{Poisson}\left(E_i \exp\left(x_i' \beta\right)\right), \text{ for } i = 1, \ldots, I$$

Development in this area has led to exploratory methods such as evaluating uniformity of risk surface associated within a region by way of a relative risk function. The implication of relative risk within a population represented scores for the average region. Focused score tests under misspecified cluster models are another aspect that is useful in the presence of prespecified sources of hazards within the disease area. This type of misspecification of score tests could mean that these were defined for one model and then applied to a different one. Proximity considered in this type of scenario is not a useful proxy to represent true exposure. Thus, selecting accurate environmental exposures and measurements is important.

3.5 Clinical trial statistics

The scope and breath of clinical trial are vast given the spectrum of trial designs available. Similarly, trial statistical issues could be a result of trial design, data monitoring, data management, data collection, and data interpretation [62]. Clinical trial statistical concepts could be challenging for nonclinical researchers or nonstatisticians to understand, despite this being fundamental to the integrity of any subsequent reports generated and published [62]. Equally, complexity of clinical trials and their data have significantly grown despite the inadequate training available, especially to clinicians [63]. West and Ficalora stipulate that over 30% of medical training does not provide sufficient statistical knowledge, based on their study. It could be argued that some nondata supported conclusions observed in peer-reviewed publications are based on empirical evidence although the limitations in statistical knowledge could be attributed as well [62–72]. Altman and colleagues reported that there is evidence that researchers apply incorrect statistical methods due to limited understanding of statistical concepts and their alignment to the research question, hypothesis, and data gathered (Table 3.5).

Adaptive clinical trials can use both Frequentist and Bayesian statistical design and analysis. There is an abundance of Bayesian adaptive design methods that are increasingly applied in a variety of clinical research studies. Bayesian statistical methods have an added advantage as these could be analysed in the presence of multiplicity relatively easily, especially in early phase dose escalation

Table 3.5 Common statistical mistakes and resolutions for these.

Statistical concern	Primary issue	Resolution
Inaccurate P-value interpretation	Overreliance of P values	Probability of observing data in accordance with the study outcomes/outcome measures is vital. Interpret P-value cut-off point of 0.05 is arbitrary and therefore should not be considered as binary statistics
Presentation of confidence intervals	Overused as a tool for assessing evidence	Confidence intervals should be used to report effect sizes inconsistent with the data. This should not be used as a replacement for a P-value
Interpreting the intent-to-treat principle clinically versus statistically	Evaluation of treatment based on optimal adherence instead of evaluation of the intervention treatment	All participants that have been randomised should be analysed, in line with the study protocol
	Mixed up between per protocol analyses and intent-to-treat	A per protocol analyses uses the population and to report the biological effect of the treatment
	Per protocol analyses reported in a trial context would mean the epidemiological comparisons are made than randomised	Avoid using statistical inference techniques where possible
	Intent-to-treat should be at the forefront when there is long-term follow up or treatment adherence is measured, even if treatment is withdrawn	Distinction between 'off-trial-drug' and 'off-trial' should be considered when the data is analysed
Missing data	Biased to treatment or treatment comparisons or treatment effect	Prevent missing data using flexible approaches to follow-up patients including removing any burdensome visits
	Difficulties to conduct intent-to-treat analyses	Alternative per protocol analyses can be completed
		Sensitivity analyses should be conducted to assess the robustness of the results if the primary endpoints were binary
Subgroup analyses interpretation	False positive results are a common issue. Interpreting a subgroup analysis in a similar manner to a sensitivity or stratified analysis is another common issue	A subgroup analysis categorises shared characteristics within a sample population and the responses to an intervention. Limit the number of subgroup analyses conducted, unless the secondary data demonstrates a high heterogeneity
Multiplicity	Lack of clarity when there are multiple hypothesis or a group of statistical inferences for a subset of parameters based on data	Multiple testing is a requirement in some clinical trials and therefore adequate statistical corrections could be useful.

Table 3.5 Common statistical mistakes and resolutions for these—cont'd

Statistical concern	Primary issue	Resolution
	gathered which produce multiple *P*-values. Multiplicity issues are more common in clinical trial data than epidemiology studies	Using PICOTA (population, intervention/comparison, outcome, timeframe and analysis) would be more useful in clinical trials than PICO (population, intervention, comparison, outcome) which would aid in prespecifying statistical approaches to adjust to the analysis plan and impact on type I and II errors
Causation versus correlation	Inability to differentiate between association in causation is common when discussing about the statistical associations between two variables. Statistical associations and clinical associations between variables can also have different meanings	Correlation is not causation from a statistical perspective. Statistically, correlation does not affirm a causation relationship and, vice versa. Avoiding assumptions and separating any analyses associated with correlation versus causation should be maintained throughout the study
Comprehensiveness of trial results	Clinical trial comprehensiveness can be different from that of an Epidemiology study. Comprehensiveness of a trial should also be aligned to the scope of the study, which should be included within the statistical analysis plan which often is lacking at the beginning of the study	Flexible approaches associated with the study design, including the statistical analysis plan should be considered. Each component of the trial should be taken into account before outcomes/outcome measures are agreed
Alignment of results to the objectives and outcome measures	The lack of alignment of outcomes to objectives as well as the study scope is a common issue in manuscripts	Ensuring the statistical tests aligned to deliberate on the predicted outcomes are important
Effective communication	Most often statistical and clinical findings are written together, or confusion arises when statistical outcomes are reported to affirm clinical outcomes and future recommendations. This isn't factually correct in many trials	Ensuring the correct use of words when describing the findings are good way to interpret and discuss the findings. Ensuring, where appropriate the statistical findings remain separate from the clinical findings is important

studies as well as seamless phase II/III trials where there is a confirmatory step involved and Umbrella or Basket clinical trials. In addition, Bayesian statistics in clinical trials are often evaluated and reported in line with the frequentist operating features such as type I error rate and as a power. Some hybrid adaptive design method could blend Frequentist and Bayesian [34,73,74] aspects, which is useful for medical device clinical trials.

Randomisation

Randomisation is considered as experimental control method used in clinical trials. The aim of randomisation is to prevent selection and accidental bias, leading to comparable groups to assign treatments and/or a treatment with a placebo. Randomisation uses the theory of probability to demonstrate the likelihood of chance when clinical trial endpoints are reported. To conduct randomisation, the process requires a schedule that can be reproduced. A randomised schedule can be generated by way of using random numbers and assigning these to subjects or conditions. Random numbers can be generated using random number tables from statistical books or software. However, software randomisation methods are used for clinical trials with large sample sizes, or the design requirement stipulates stratified or restricted randomisation. There are a number of techniques used for clinical trial randomisation as stipulated below:

- Simple randomisation: This is a single sequence random assignment method where complete randomness is maintained throughout the experiment. It is a commonly used method and considered to be a basic technique used in two-arm clinical trials where a control versus a treatment is tested. The method can be used with any sample size although it could be problematic with unequal participants across arms.
- Block or cluster randomisation: This is a method used to randomise patients into groups [75,76]. The clusters are small and maintain a balanced sample size with a predefined group assignment. Clusters are determined based on the research question, sample size, and operationalisation required to recruit participants [76]. The effective use of cluster randomisation would be with smaller increments where these can be efficiently controlled. However, if the statistical analysis plan for the study requires comparing covariates. For example, one group may have more participants with confounders that could negatively influence the results. Managing these covariates is important to help with a comprehensive interpretation. Any potential bias that is detected should be further explored to justify the findings to prevent the power of the clinical trial.
- Stratified randomisation: This method is used to manage the covariates and their influence. The technique could achieve balanced baseline characteristics and report the potential relationship shared between covariates and the dependent variables. The process of stratified randomisation is complete by way of developing a separate block for combinations of covariates where participants are allocated to the block. Stratified

randomisation could balance the treatment and control groups for age or sex and works well for trials with small sample sizes. However, a significant limitation with this technique is that it can only be applicable when all participants are in the clinical trial.

- Covariate adaptive randomisation: This method is a fairly new method and is considered as an alternative randomisation method [77,78]. The process with this technique would be to sequentially assign a patient to a treatment group based on the covariates and prior participant assignments. This method uses a minimisation approach by way of evaluating the imbalance of sample size using multiple covariates. Imbalance of covariates is an issue that could negatively impact the interpretation of the results [78].

Sensitivity analysis

The sensitivity analysis is important to understand the probabilistic outcomes that are often calculated in clinical trials and epidemiology studies. Specificity and sensitivity are key facets within sample sizes where demographics and/or disease characteristics could be better assessed. These can be evaluated along with comparing interventions. A simple and linear mathematical equation to assess sensitivity and specificity is as follows:

$$\text{Sensitivity} = \frac{\text{S.Pr} \times \text{T}+}{\text{D}+} \quad \text{Specificity} = \frac{\text{S.Pr} \times \text{T}-}{\text{D}-}$$

Sensitivity probability—S.Pr.
Disease positive—D+.
Positive test—T+.
Negative test—T−.

The common terms for sensitivity and specificity could be expressed in a mathematical equation as shown below and a contingency (Table 3.6).

$$\text{Sensitivity} = \frac{\text{TP}}{\text{TP} + \text{FN}}$$

$$\text{Specificity} = \frac{\text{TN}}{\text{TN} + \text{FP}}$$

TP = True positive
TN = True negative
FP = False positive
FN = False negative

Table 3.6 A contingency table for the above mathematical equation.

| | | Disease | |
		Positive	Negative
Test	Negative	False negative	True negative
	Positive	True positive	False positive
Control	Neutral	True positive	True negative
	Neutral	True positive	True negative

Table 3.6: These parameters quantify the validity of a test when it is evaluated in a population that represents the spectrum of patients in whom it would be logical and clinically useful to use the test. The most obvious limitation of evaluating a screening test is identifying an optimal gold standard to determine the disease status. In the evaluation of new screening tests, existing tests are often used as the gold standard. Disagreement or poor sensitivity and specificity of the new test could mean that the new test does not work as well as, or that it is actually superior to, the existing test. A histological test from a biopsy is the least disputable gold standard. Nonetheless, the limitation with regard to the gold standard is unavoidable and must be recognised in the continuous evaluation of clinical screening and diagnostic testing.

Case study

Exploring *bidirectional* clinical relationships can be complex especially where the statistical and inferences can be different. This is equally complex if the bidirectionality is between a physical and mental health conditions. Often there is a lack of knowledge between the longitudinal and reciprocal relationship clinically due to the large number of symptoms that are difficult to delineate between the conditions. This is an important feature for clinicians who need to use this information to evaluate the impact of the findings on patient care and future research. A good example of this is the ELEMI project's Gestational Diabetes systematic review and metaanalysis [79]. The mental health assessments used for the purpose of the metaanalysis are indicated in Table 3.7.

Learning objectives

- Studies were categorised as per characteristics and synthesised based on relative risks (RRs), odds ratios (ORs), prevalence

Table 3.7 The mental health assessments used in the metaanalyses.

Mental health questionnaires	Scale	Relevance to BAME population
CES-D	0–3; 0 = rarely or none of the time, 1 = some or little of the time, 2 = moderately or much of the time and 3 = most or almost all of the time	Has been adapted to the Korean version (CES-D-K) this was reliable and valid for Korean [80] and Armenian population [81] CES-D Cronbach's $\alpha = 0.825$ indicative of high internal reliability in Bolivian patients [82]. In South Africa the 10 item version was validated in the Zulu, Xhosa and Afrikaans population [83] ($\alpha = 0.69$–0.89), and adequate concurrent validity
BSI	Items are scored on a 5-point Likert scale, ranging from 0 ('not at all') to 4 ('extremely')	Been tested over 400 studies, with nonwhite sample ranging between 15% in nonclinical adult population, 33% in clinical population, 44% in inpatients and 42% in adolescent non clinical population therefore has reliability and validity
EPDS	Scores of 10–12 represent borderline and 0–9 not depressed	Used in Caribbean women with Perinatal depression [84] Also validated in Nigerian women [85]
DASS-21	Respondents rate items on a 0 ('did not apply to me at all') to 3 ('applied to me very much/most of the time').	Yes
BDI-II	Each item is rated on a 4 point scale ranging from 0 to 3 and has a total score of 63 Ranges 0–13 minimal; 14–19 mild; 20–28 moderate and 29–63 severe depressive symptoms	Outpatient sample had 4% (21) African American and Asian American 4% (18) and Hispanic 1% However, has validity and is widely used in psychiatry

risks (PRs), media, mean differences (MDs), and their 95%CI were collated as part of the data synthesis method.

- Prevalence tables were generated to show the subgroup categories of ethnicity, race, and geographical location.
- Potential barriers were reported using a narrative approach using themes.
- Studies that reported RR were categorised using the formulae below to determine the adjusted and unadjusted analysis. The term adjusted analysis is based upon the adjusted and crude

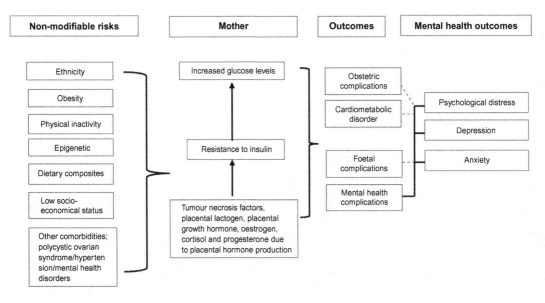

Fig. 3.10 A causation tree developed based on evidence produced.

OR. P_0 was considered as the general prevalence of GDM within the context of pregnant woman. The quantitative data were metaanalysed using predefined variables.

$$\hat{RR} = \frac{OR}{1 - P_0 + P_0 * OR}$$

- Heterogeneity was assessed using I^2
- Publication bias was assessed using Egger's test
- A causation tree was demonstrated based on the evidence synthesised (Fig. 3.10)

References

[1] Irgens LM. The roots of Norwegian epidemiology—Norwegian epidemiology in the 19th century. Nor Epidemiol 2015;25(1–2). https://doi.org/10.5324/nje.v25i1-2.1885.

[2] Kiaer A-N. Statistische Beitraege zur Beleuchtung der ehelichen Fruchtbarkeit (Études statistiques s1w la (écondité tfes mariages). Christiania: Jacob Dybwad; 1903.

[3] Galimberti E, Manzini F, Riva MA. Bernardino Ramazzini (1633-1714): an often forgotten pioneer in maritime health. Int Marit Health 2014;65(1):41. https://doi.org/10.5603/MH.2014.0009. 24677127.

[4] Meitzen A, Falkner RP. History, theory, and technique of statistics. Part first: history of statistics. Ann Am Acad Pol Soc Sci 1891;1:1–100. JSTOR http://www.jstor.org/stable/1008943. [Accessed 21 July 2022].

[5] Morabia A. Pierre-Charles-Alexandre Louis and the evaluation of bloodletting. J R Soc Med 2006;99(3):158–60. https://doi.org/10.1258/jrsm.99.3.158.

[6] Bradshaw NA. Florence Nightingale (1820–1910): an unexpected master of data. Patterns (N Y) 2020;1(2):100036. Published 2020 May 8 https://doi.org/10.1016/j.patter.2020.100036.

[7] Sheynin OB. On the history of medical statistics. Arch Hist Exact Sci 1982;26:241–86. (46 pages), Springer.

[8] Bolstad WM. Bayesian inference for Poisson. In: Introduction to Bayesian statistics. Hoboken, NJ: John Wiley & Sons; 2007. p. 183–98. 67.

[9] Ghosh M, Natarajan K, Waller LA, Kim D. Hierarchical Bayes GLMs for the analysis of spatial data: an application to disease mapping. J Stat Plan Inference 1999;75(2):305–18.

[10] Devine OJ, Louis TA, Halloran ME. Empirical Bayes methods for stabilizing incidence rates before mapping. Epidemiology 1994;5(6):622–30.

[11] Delanerolle GK, Shetty S, Raymont V. A perspective: use of machine learning models to predict the risk of multimorbidity. LOJ Med Sci 2022;5(5):574–9.

[12] Clayton D, Kaldor J. Empirical Bayes estimates of age-standardised relative risks for use in disease mapping. Biometrics 1987;43(3):671–81.

[13] Cressie N, Read TRC. Spatial data analysis of regional counts. Biom J 1989;6:699–719.

[14] Ghosh JK, Delampady M, Samanta T. An introduction to Bayesian analysis: theory and methods. New York, NY: Springer; 2006.

[15] Louis TA, Shen W. Innovations in Bayes and empirical Bayes methods: estimating parameters, populations and ranks. Stat Med 1999;18(17–18):2493–505.

[16] Maiti T. Hierarchical Bayes estimation of mortality rates for disease mapping. J Stat Plan Inference 1998;69(2):339–48.

[17] Greco FP, Lawson AB, Cocchi D, Temples T. Some interpolation estimators in environmental risk assessment for spatially misaligned health data. Environ Ecol Stat 2005;12(4):379–95.

[18] Besag J, York J, Mollie A. Bayesian image restoration, with two applications in spatial statistics. Ann Inst Stat Math 1991;43:1–59.

[19] Kim H, Sun DC, Tsutakawa RK. Lognormal vs. gamma: extra variations. Biom J 2002;44(3):305–23.

[20] Bell BS, Broemeling LD. A Bayesian analysis for spatial processes with application to disease mapping. Stat Med 2000;19(7):957–74.

[21] Ocana-Riola R. The misuse of count data aggregated over time for disease mapping. Stat Med 2007;26(24):4489–504.

[22] Gelfand AE, Vounatsou P. Proper multivariate conditional autoregressive models for spatial data analysis. Biostatistics 2003;4(1):11–25.

[23] Davey Smith G, Ebrahim S. 'Mendelian randomization': can genetic epidemiology contribute to understanding environmental determinants of disease? Int J Epidemiol 2003;32:1–22.

[24] Burgess S, Thompson SG. Mendelian randomization: methods for using genetic variants in causal estimation. Boca Raton, FL: Chapman & Hall; 2015.

[25] Davey Smith G, Hemani G. Mendelian randomization: genetic anchors for causal inference in epidemiological studies. Hum Mol Genet 2014;23(R1): R89–98. https://doi.org/10.1093/hmg/ddu328.

[26] Burgess S, Butterworth A, Malarstig A, Thompson SG. Use of Mendelian randomisation to assess potential benefit of clinical intervention. BMJ 2012;345: e7325. https://doi.org/10.1136/bmj.e7325.

[27] Takagi S, Baba S, Iwai N, et al. The aldehyde dehydrogenase 2 gene is a risk factor for hypertension in Japanese but does not alter the sensitivity to pressor effects of alcohol: the Suita study. Hypertens Res 2001;24:365–70. https://doi.org/10.1291/hypres.24.365.

[28] Chen L, Davey Smith G, Harbord RM, Lewis SJ. Alcohol intake and blood pressure: a systematic review implementing a Mendelian randomization

approach. PLoS Med 2008;5:e52. https://doi.org/10.1371/journal.pmed.0050052.

[29] Hernán M, Robins J. Causal inference. Chapman & Hall/CRC; 2018.

[30] Burgess S, Thompson SG. Mendelian randomization: methods for using genetic variants in causal estimation. Boca Raton: CRC Press, Taylor & Francis Group; 2015.

[31] Hausman JA. Specification tests in econometrics. Econometrica 1978;46:1251–71. https://doi.org/10.2307/1913827.

[32] Altman DG, Bland JM. Interaction revisited: the difference between two estimates. BMJ 2003;326:219. https://doi.org/10.1136/bmj.326.7382.219.

[33] Angrist JD, Pischke JS. Mostly harmless econometrics: an empiricist's companion. Princeton University Press; 2008.

[34] Stallard N, Whitehead J, Cleall S. Decision-making in a phase II clinical trial: a new approach combining Bayesian and frequentist concepts. Pharm Stat 2005;4:119–28. https://doi.org/10.1002/pst.164.

[35] Kroeger A, Lenhart A, Ochoa M, Villegas E, Levy M, Alexander N, et al. Effective control of dengue vectors with curtains and water container covers treated with insecticide in Mexico and Venezuela: cluster ran- domised trials. BMJ 2006;332:1247–52.

[36] Banerjee S, Carlin BP, Gelfrand AE. Hierarchical modeling and analysis for spatial data. Boca Raton: Chapman & Hall/CRC; 2015.

[37] Lenhart A, Orelus N, Maskill R, Alexander N, Streit T, McCall PJ. Insecticide-treated bednets to control dengue vectors: preliminary evidence from a controlled trial in Haiti. Tropical Med Int Health 2008;13:56–67.

[38] Miguel E, Kremer M. Worms: identifying impacts on education and health in the presence of treatment externalities. Econometrica 2004;72:159–217.

[39] Ali M, Thiem VD, Park JK, Ochiai RL, Canh DG, Danovaro-Holliday MC, et al. Geographic analysis of vaccine uptake in a cluster-randomized controlled trial in Hue, Vietnam. Health Place 2007;13:577–87.

[40] Chao DL, Park JK, Marks F, Ochiai RL, Longini IM, Halloran ME. The contribution of neighbours to an individual's risk of typhoid outcome. Epidemiol Infect 2015;143:3520–7.

[41] Guindo A, Sagara I, Ouedraogo B, et al. Spatial heterogeneity of environmental risk in randomized prevention trials: consequences and modeling. BMC Med Res Methodol 2019;19:149. https://doi.org/10.1186/s12874-019-0759-z.

[42] Alexander ND, Moyeed RA, Hyun PJ, Dimber ZB, Bockarie MJ, Stander J, et al. Spatial variation of Anopheles-transmitted Wuchereria bancrofti and Plasmodium falciparum infection densities in Papua New Guinea. Filaria J 2003;2:14.

[43] Moran PAP. Notes on continuous stochastic phenomena. Biometrika 1950;37 (1–2):17–23.

[44] Geary RC. The contiguity ratio and statistical mapping. Inc Stat 1954;5 (3):115–46.

[45] Anselin L. Local indicators of spatial association—LISA. Geogr Anal 1995;27 (2):93–115.

[46] Kulldorff M, Song C, Gregorio D, Samociuk H, DeChello L. Cancer map patterns: are they random or not? Am J Prev Med 2006;30(2 Suppl):S37–49.

[47] Tango T. A test for spatial disease clustering adjusted for multiple testing. Stat Med 2000;19(2):191–204.

[48] Kulldorff M. A spatial scan statistic. Commun Stat Theory Methods 1997;26 (6):1481–96.

[49] Elliott P, Wartenberg D. Spatial epidemiology: current approaches and future challenges. Environ Health Perspect 2004;112(9):998–1006.

[50] Lai P-C, So F-M, Chan K-W. Spatial epidemiological approaches in disease mapping and analysis. Baton Rouge: CRC Press; 2008.

[51] Shen W, Louis TA. Triple-goal estimates for disease mapping. Stat Med 2000;19 (17–18):2295–308.

[52] Inskip H, Beral V, Fraser P, Haskey J. Methods for age-adjustment of rates. Stat Med 1983;2(4):455–66.

[53] Anselin L. Under the hood. Issues in the specification and interpretation of spatial regression models. Agric Econ 2002;27(3):247–67.

[54] Bavaud F. Models for spatial weights: a systematic look. Geogr Anal 1998;30 (2):153–71.

[55] Cliff AD, Ord JK. Spatial processes: models and applications. London: Pion; 1981.

[56] Anselin L, Lozano N, Koschinsky J. Rate transformations and smoothing. Urbana, IL: Department of Geography, University of Illinois; 2006.

[57] Waller LA, Gotway CA. Applied spatial statistics for public health data. Chichester: John Wiley & Sons; 2004.

[58] Ausner JS, Kramer S. Epidemiology: an introductory text. Philadelphia: W.B. Saunders; 1985.

[59] Disease mapping and risk assessment for public health decision-making. Report on a WHO workshop 1999 European Health21 Target 10, 19, www. efaidnbmnnnibpcajpcglclefindmkaj/, https://apps.who.int/iris/bitstream/ handle/10665/108152/E63686.pdf?sequence=1&isAllowed=y. [Accessed 2 July 2022].

[60] Wagner M, Robinson J, Tsui F, et al. Design of a national retail data monitor for public health surveillance. J Am Med Inform Assoc 2003;10:409–18.

[61] Waller LA, Carlin BP. Disease mapping. In: Chapman & Hall/CRC handbooks of modern statistical methods, vol. 2010; 2010. p. 217–43. https://doi.org/ 10.1201/9781420072884-c14. 25285319. PMCID: PMC4180601.

[62] Altman DG, Bland JM. Absence of evidence is not evidence of absence. BMJ 1995;311:485. https://doi.org/10.1136/bmj.311.7003.485.

[63] Wulff HR, Andersen B, Brandenhoff P, Guttler F. What do doctors know about statistics? Stat Med 1986;6:3–10. https://doi.org/10.1002/sim.4780060103.

[64] Altman DG. Statistical reviewing for medical journals. Stat Med 1998;17:2661–74. https://doi.org/10.1002/(sici)1097-0258(19981215)17:23% 3C2661::aid-sim33%3E3.0.co;2-b.

[65] Altman DG, Bland JM. Improving doctors' understanding of statistics. J R Stat Soc Ser A 1998;154:223–67. https://doi.org/10.2307/2983040.

[66] Berwick D, Fineber HV, Weinstein MC. When doctors meet numbers. Am J Med 1981;71:991–8. https://doi.org/10.1016/0002-9343(81)90325-9.

[67] Gardner MJ, Altman DG. Confidence intervals rather than P-values: estimation rather than hypothesis testing. BMJ 1986;292:746–50. https://doi.org/ 10.1136/bmj.292.6522.746.

[68] Glantz SA. How to detect, correct and prevent errors in the medical literature. Biostatistics 1980;61:1–7. https://doi.org/10.1161/01.cir.61.1.1.

[69] Horton NJ, Switzer SS. Statistical methods in the journal (letter). N Engl J Med 2005;353:1977–9. https://doi.org/10.1056/nejm200511033531823.

[70] Weiss ST, Samet JM. An assessment of physician knowledge of epidemiology and biostatistics. J Med Educ 1980;55:692–7. https://doi.org/ 10.1097/00001888-198008000-00007.

[71] West CP, Ficalora RD. Clinician attitudes towards biostatistics. Mayo Clin Proc 2007;82:939–43. https://doi.org/10.4065/82.8.939.

[72] Windish DM, Huot SJ, Free ML. Medicine residents' understanding of the biostatistics and results in the medical literature. JAMA 2007;298:1010–22. https://doi.org/10.1001/jama.298.9.1010.

[73] Campbell G. Similarities and differences of Bayesian designs and adaptive designs for medical devices: a regulatory view. Stat Biopharm Res 2013;5:356–68. https://doi.org/10.1080/19466315.2013.846873.

[74] Hartley AM. Adaptive blinded sample size adjustment for comparing two normal means-a mostly Bayesian approach. Pharm Stat 2012;11:230–40. https://doi.org/10.1002/pst.538.

[75] Lachin JM, Matis JP, Wei LJ. Randomizations in clinical trails, conclusions and recommendations. Control Clin Trails 1988;9:365–74.

[76] Suresh K. An overview of randomization techniques: an unbiased assessment of outcome in clinical research. J Hum Reprod Sci 2011;4(1):8–11. https://doi.org/10.4103/0974-1208.82352.

[77] Zalene M. Randomized consent designs for clinical trails: an update. Stat Med 1990;9:645–56.

[78] Fleiss JL, Levin B, Park MC. A statistical methods for rates and proportion. 3rd ed. Hoboken, NJ: John Wiley and Sons; 2003.

[79] Delanerolle G, Phiri P, Zeng Y, Marston K, Tempest N, Busuulwa P, Shetty A, Goodison W, Muniraman H, Duffy G, Elliot K, Maclean A, Majumder K, Hirsch M, Rathod S, Raymont V, Shi JQ, Hapangama DK. A systematic review and meta-analysis of gestational diabetes mellitus and mental health among BAME populations. EClinicalMedicine 2021;38:101016. https://doi.org/10.1016/j.eclinm.2021.101016. 34308317. PMCID: PMC8283332.

[80] Cho MJ, Kim KH. Use of the center for epidemiologic studies depression (CES-D) scale in Korea. J Nerv Ment Dis 1998;186(5):304–10. https://doi.org/10.1097/00005053-199805000-00007. 9612448.

[81] Demirchyan A, Petrosyan V, Thompson ME. Psychometric value of the center for epidemiologic studies depression (CES-D) scale for screening of depressive symptoms in Armenian population. J Affect Disord 2011;133(3):489–98. https://doi.org/10.1016/j.jad.2011.04.042. Epub 2011 May 23 21601288.

[82] Schantz K, Reighard C, Aikens JE, Aruquipa A, Pinto B, Valverde H, et al. Screening for depression in Andean Latin America: factor structure and reliability of the CES-D short form and the PHQ-8 among Bolivian public hospital patients. Int J Psychiatry Med 2017;52(4–6):315–27.

[83] Baron EC, Davies T, Lund C. Validation of the 10-item centre for epidemiological studies depression scale (CES-D-10) in Zulu, Xhosa and Afrikaans populations in South Africa. BMC Psychiatry 2017;17(1):6. https://doi.org/10.1186/s12888-016-1178-x. 28068955. PMCID: PMC5223549.

[84] Edge D, Baker D, Rogers A. Perinatal depression among black Caribbean women. Health Soc Care Community 2004;12:430–8.

[85] Uwakwe R. Affective (depressive) morbidity in puerperal Nigerian women: validation of the Edinburgh postnatal depression scale. Acta Psychiatr Scand 2003. https://doi.org/10.1034/j.1600-0447.2003.02477.x. 2003.

4

Research ethics and supporting evolving research

Key messages

- Scientific concepts and the clinical relevance must be aligned to ensure ethical conduct of any resulting research.
- Ensuring participant rights remain protected during the ethical conduct of research is an important facet to consider.
- All staff associated with setting up and delivering research require a comprehensive understanding of research ethics.
- Relevant training should be provided to all research staff to ensure ethical practices are maintained throughout the conduct of research.

4.1 Introduction

Research ethics is defined primarily as a code of professional conduct which all researchers are held up to. Ethical conduct of clinical research is paramount to develop new interventions and knowledge for improving health and care with evidence-based approaches that are safe and show effectiveness. Much of the knowledge we have today about the therapeutic interventions and treatment has been investigated through clinical trials that generate high-quality evidence about the safety and efficacy. Learning ethical norms happens throughout the lifespan of mankind. The influence of a person's home environment, religion, school, and social setting impacts their sense of right and wrong. Development of the human mind throughout life would equally impact the ethical views and practices observed as ethical norms are ubiquitous. Despite there being an argument for ethical behaviour being common sense, Good Clinical Practice (GCP) underpinned by regulations demonstrates a code of practice that is also ethically aligned to conducting research. The concept of GCP was put together following the Nuremberg Code which is a legal and ethical principle that was affirmed following the trial

Clinical Trials and Tribulations. https://doi.org/10.1016/B978-0-12-821787-0.00011-8

of the Nazi doctors following World War II. This event has been considered as an authoritative legal reference for human experimentation without consent. The principles of GCP are based on natural laws of human rights, which are covered within the Declaration of Helsinki which is the most well-known medical research guideline. This is an official policy within the World Medical Association that was adopted in 1964. Undoubtedly, this policy document has been revised many times to balance the need to generate clinical knowledge to meet the healthcare interests of the global population. Key facets to consider when assessing ethical standards in addition to the code of practice for ethics are demonstrated in Fig. 4.1.

Research ethics in the real world is another consideration that needs to be reflected on, especially with increasing pressures and to ensure researchers from academia and healthcare professionals deliver effectively. In a climate where competitiveness at its peak for securing grants, fulfilling planned sample sizes, and completing all milestones in a timely manner within the specified budget, ethical practices could often be forgotten. A key feature that should be considered is the application of research ethics in real-world research that is beyond the scope of the individual, social norms including the digital sense [1], professional, political,

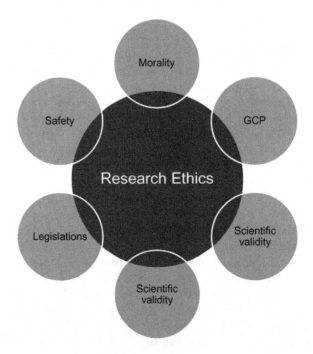

Fig. 4.1 Key components of ethical standards.

and institutional policies, as well as indigenous or traditions of Euro-Western research. Until the 1970s or so, clinical research in many parts of the world where the legitimacy of the protocol along and with an institutional approval was considered as the sole authority. Protecting patients have always been warranted by the commitment of clinicians, by the Hippocratic Oath '*to do no harm*'. The requirement of research ethics and medical ethics emerged where research misconduct became apparent. Clinical research often confronts clinicians with ethical dilemmas, especially given professional ethics can be intertwined with the obligation to do or not do a procedure to benefit patients. The distinction between research and clinical ethics around human experimentation can often be a trade-off for current patient benefit and scientific progress to optimise healthcare for future patient, respectively.

Clinical trials are a global phenomenon that now reach a much more diverse group of participants than decades ago, where the number of patients taking part increases yearly. All stages of conducting research are now better documented through processes and formulations of data gathering as well as their reporting. It is encouraged to publish any negative research results which were often omitted decades ago. This paradigmal shift has meant change management and leadership are required to maintain ethical approaches whilst still delivering research in a rapidly evolving world. Historically, the ethical problem of clinical trials stems from the '*risk and burden*' concept to participants. There has been much debate around the use of placebos when testing a novel intervention to assess efficacy and effectiveness. Placebos have been associated with deception and the contentious notion of *harm* to those patients who do not receive a treatment when they are ill. Placebo use among patients with chronic conditions could result in death although in such circumstances, it would be deemed unethical. An added complication would be that the limitation of this ethical view means further development of treatments for future patients who have the same chronic condition. This does provide an opportunity to evolve novel methods and methodologies in clinical trials to address other avenues to still develop and further the scientific landscape. An example of this would be the use of crossover trials where the patient could move from a predetermined time point from one arm to another despite being given a placebo initially, and vice versa. Another ethical and scientifically viable method is the 'ad-on' trial design where patients in both arms would be provided standard treatment plus the novel intervention or the placebo. This prevents the patient from not receiving a treatment, thereby still adhering to the '*to do no harm*'.

In addition, the changing global population and subsequent healthcare demands require research ethics to be applied pre- and post-clinical trials. In particular, in the case of drug trials where the therapies are provided for the duration of the trial than the life-course of the patient. Whilst some patients and healthcare systems may be able to afford treatments if they are improving a patient's condition, others may not have the financial stability to continue with these once a trial has completed. The ethical implications these scenarios raise do not have a straightforward and simple solution. As such, at the point that trials are designed and budgeted and considerations are made for site selection, ethical practices should be considered. This invaluable step could support the reduction of disparities when accessing novel therapies.

Key components assessed by Research Ethics Committees (REC) include if stress, discomfort, or risk to participants both physically and mentally is posed from the research studies proposed. Imperative factors for RECs include clinical benefit to the patient versus the risk posed by a novel intervention. As such, researchers would be expected to demonstrate measures to reduce the risk, as well as evidence to protect participant rights. This is particularly important for vulnerable populations such as those with a disability or children. Hence, RECs may require additional documentation describing measures such as informed consent forms for parents and/or legal guardians.

4.2 Morality versus ethics

Ethics and morality are a problematic divide given the variability observed in philosophical and social roles. Moral life driven by moral theory can cover both a person's moral and ethical experience as this could be pervasive.

Modern moral philosophy

Revisiting the Greece of Socrates, Plato, and Aristotle, Raws in 2005, made a brief separation between modern and classical moral philosophy in order to elucidate the idea of complex formation of a certain moral conception [2]. From a more radical perspective, Elizabeth Anscombe, in 1958, defended the idea that we should not think and analyse moral philosophy before understanding the concepts of obligation and moral duty, that is, what is morally right and wrong. Anscombe begins her argument by directing our attention to the difference between modern moral philosophising and the kind of ethical reflection that we find in

Aristotle [3]. On the other hand, in a rationalist conception, moral philosophy is the knowledge of motivations and intentions (which move the moral subject internally) and of the means and ends of moral action capable of realising those motivations and intentions.

According to Anscombe, the landscape of modern moral philosophy (i.e. those since Butler) is stated as moral concepts, such as 'ought', which have now lost the context within which they once made sense. There is the use of the term 'duty' – and what we might call 'non-moral duty' – which relates directly to non-moral goodness or badness. For example, 'This engine needs oil' means something like 'this engine is running without oil and could be damaged' [4,5] Managed recovery (pausing non-essential research to prioritise Covid-19-related research). Impact on patients affected by trials that were paused.

Moral injury and its important when assessing research ethics

From a legal point of view, the concept of damage can be understood in its physical dimension or in a moral sense. Currently, laws protect the physical integrity and property of people, especially in the field of research and clinical trials. However, there are issues that we still cannot fully understand. For instance, issues related to feelings and prestige. In order for this underdeveloped field to be legally protected, we resort to moral damages. Moral damage can still be understood as a strong emotional response that can occur after an event that violate a person's moral or ethical code. Potentially morally harmful events include the individuals themselves or their acts of omission (or commission). As a clear example, we can use healthcare workers that do not receive adequate protective equipment, or that are obligated to work more hours than they are used to or were mandated by law [6–20].

Therefore, based on moral and ethical tenets, i.e. when and how to correctly make a decision while minimising harm, there is a strong link between what is morally correct and decision-making. All decision-making in the clinical environment must be guided by morally and ethically (also conventionally) accepted principles in order to minimise damages.

Decision theory

Medicine in general, expanding this vision to the entire area of health, lives in eternal confrontation in the search for decision-making with maximum precision in scenarios of uncertainty. These uncertain scenarios unfold in various forms: the first source of uncertainty being the patient. The second major source of uncertainty lies in the results coming from technologies that are not used in the medical field, such as the results of complementary exams. The third source of uncertainty is found again in the human element. This time in the figure of the doctor. From this perspective, the diagnoses that are made, and from which the therapeutic decisions are based, have presented great variability and unreliable results. Systems that support clinical diagnosis that are based on decision theory can be very useful in clinical settings, for the use of these systems tends to reduce inaccuracies in a subtle but very important way.

Decision theory has been used as a tool to act logically and concisely in situations where outcomes are inconsistent or uncertain. It is an effective tool that helps in decision-making and that takes into account (after careful deliberation) a logical sequence of what is wanted, what is known, and what can be done [7–9].

Through an ethical and moral lens, following the moral dilemma, decision theory must always be based on circumstances where any final decision does not cause any other harm. In general, the criterion used to resolve a dilemma or make an important decision in the face of what is still not known is always the decision that causes the least harm, following the line of non-maleficence found in the precepts of bioethics.

Logical positivism

Logical positivism, later known as logical empiricism, was a movement in Western philosophy that advocated the verification principle [10]. Throughout the 1930s, it gained strength in Europe, and its main objective was to avoid unclear language and unverifiable or scientifically based statements, converting philosophy into scientific philosophy [11]. Logical positivism dominated not only disease tracking, but epidemiology and medical research in general, to the point of defending the idea that scientific research is the only way to investigate disease phenomena. However [12], logical positivism has become erroneously stereotyped as a movement to regulate the scientific process and set rigid standards for it.

Logical empiricism

After World War II, the movement shifted to a milder variant called logical empiricism. According to Salmon, a fundamental principle of logical empiricism is that the guarantee for all scientific knowledge rests on empirical evidence together with logic [13]. Logical empiricism was a dynamic form of philosophy based on mathematical and physical foundations, which became one of the main references in the philosophy of science. Furthermore, it played a major role in analytical philosophy, which is an important facet to consider when writing and reviewing research protocols. The logical state can often shift based on gathered data and synthesis of the evidence.

Traditionalism

Traditionalism can be defined as a philosophical and political system, also called classical conservatism or traditional conservatism, which places tradition as a criterion and rule [14] for decision-making. However, traditionalists differ from conservatives in that they are not averse to social, political, group, or individual innovations. While the conservative wants to maintain the existing social, political, and economic order, the traditionalist is more sensitive to change. Even though they are different, the traditionalist movement still shows some resistance in adhering to the new, such as the advancement of technology in science. Still in the 21st century, after the Revolution 4.0 (the 4th Industrial Revolution), resistance of the technological transition in the health area is still notorious.

4.3   Evolving research ethics

Research ethics continues to evolve with sociological influences, growing healthcare, and population demands. There is a fundamental shift especially in the era of COVID-19 where peer review includes research design, methodologies, and transition of these to research practice. Flexibility in peer review was a key factor that raised debates among clinicians, researchers, and the public. Adaptations to procedural assessments for interventions being developed, quality of interventions, and the unprecedented need to protect human life were all valuable factors to consider. These were catalysts for scholars and the lay personal in ethics committees to consider as most COVID-19 interventions were *disruptive* interventions which continue to evolve and influence non-communicable diseases [15]. The pandemic opened a window of opportunity to rethink ethical practices and it's adaptation to develop flexible models of research. The shift in mindset continues to influence methodologies and study delivery mechanisms whilst sustaining adherence to highest ethical and research standards.

The shift from *unprepared* to *prepared* has already commenced with innovative ways to maintain the current shift. For example, the continued use of digital [16] platforms and scholarly activities in clinical research to improve transparency, informativeness, and social value has introduced research participant follow-up procedures to be conducted remotely. During the pre-COVID era, follow-up procedures were primarily conducted face to face, and telephone discussions were rare [17,18]. Rethinking and rearticulating the knowledge production process has allowed everyone to evaluate partnerships and revisit the completion of research inquiries to optimise clinical practice. To enable continuous improvement in clinical and research practices, discussions around ethical implications should continue. The pursuit of therapeutic benefit for all patients in an ethical manner should be the ultimate goal to sustain clinical research.

Case study

The Duff report brings to light a variety of procedural issues such as risk assessments during the conduct of the TGN1412 drug trial that was sponsored by Paraxel and conducted at the Northwick Park hospital. The Duff report was led by Professor Gordon Duff and setup by the Health Secretary of the United Kingdom at the time, Patricia Hewitt.

The issues of this trial led to significant legislative and process changes to conduct clinical trials. Many have debated around the ethical implications associated with the availability of carefully constructed risk assessments, especially for first-in-man studies. In the United Kingdom, risk assessments are now conducted by study sponsors to ensure preventative measures and risk mitigation plans are put in place prior to the initiation of a study. Many have argued the ethics committee approved the trial protocol used to test TGN1412 and multiorgan failure demonstrated in the patients were unexpected, thereby the conduct of the study was ethically appropriate. Ethical implications to the participants still require expert advice, especially when a team is conducting a high-risk study. A more comprehensive review should have been undertaken, including but not limited to identifying if there was any evidence synthesis conducted to better understand adverse reactions to new drugs. A key recommendation from the Duff report was the use of unpublished or abandoned trial information to better understand adverse reactions to new drugs and that this task should be done by universities, hospitals, and industry. In other words, a systematic approach to including this information in a study protocol would be useful. In addition, the litigation team of the two men that were injured due to the TGN1412 drug pointed out the change in legislations around safe doses for human use was an important factor to determine. However, the purpose of conducting a first-in-human clinical trial is to determine the safety doses for human use. This is a complex ethical component to address especially when taking into account immune responses differ across people. However, this does not negate the notion of protecting the rights and wellbeing of trial participants should be considered at the point of securing ethical approvals.

Learning objectives

It is important to conduct high-quality scientifically and ethically justifiable research. This implies to all processes and procedures conducted throughout the clinical trial and/or study life cycle.

1. Risk averse thinking is important for ethics committees to consider when assessing studies to ensure the designed risk mitigation plans are ethically justifiable.
2. There is more information available now due to the conduct of a high volume of clinical trials, increased participation of patients in clinical research studies, improved gathering of adverse reaction data including information on immune responses, and scientific advancement to better predict safety profiles of novel drugs. The subsequent availability of data for evidence synthesis and their availability to ethics committees is useful to make more informed decisions

References

[1] Phiri P, Cavalini H, Shetty S, Delanerolle G. Digital maturity consulting and strategizing to optimise services: an overview. J Med Internet Res 2022;, 37545. https://doi.org/10.2196/preprints.37545.

[2] Rawls J. História da filosofia moral. Martins Fontes: São Paulo; 2005.

[3] Royal Institute of Philosophy. Royal Institute of Philosophy supplement 87, A centenary celebration: Anscombe, foot, Midgley, and Murdoch; 2019.

[4] Anscombe GEM. Modern moral philosophy repr. in Crisp and Slote; 1997. p. 26–44. Orig pub Philosophy 1997, 33, 1–19.

[5] Aristotle. In: Bywater J, editor. Ethica Nicomachea (EN). Oxford: Clarendon Press; 1894.

[6] Litz BT, Stein N, Delaney E, Lebowitz L, Nash WP, Silva C, et al. Moral injury and moral repair in war veterans: a preliminary model and intervention strategy. Clin Psychol Rev 2009;29:695–706. https://doi.org/10.1016/j.cpr.2009.07.003.

[7] Berger JO. Statistical decision theory and Baysian analysis. New York: Springer; 1985.

[8] Keeney RL, Raiffa H. Decisions with multiple objectives. John Wiley & Sons; 1976.

[9] de Souza FMC, de Souza BC, da Silva AS. Elementos da Pesquisa Científica em Medicina. Recife: Editora Universitária da Universidade Federal de Pernambuco; 2002.

[10] Godfrey-Smith P. Theory and reality: an introduction to the philosophy of science. Chicago: University of Chicago Press; 2010.

[11] Friedman M. Reconsidering logical positivism. New York: Cambridge University Press; 1999.

[12] Mayer JD. Challenges to understanding spatial patterns of disease: philosophical alternatives to logical positivism. Soc Sci Med 1992;35(4):579–87. https://doi.org/10.1016/0277-9536(92)90351-p.

[13] Salmon WC. Logical Empiricism. W H Newton-Smith; 2017. https://doi.org/10.1002/9781405164481.ch36.

[14] Japiassú H, Marcondes D. Basic dictionary of philosophy. Rio de Janeiro: Zahar; 1993.

[15] Chau SWH, Wong OWH, Ramakrishnan R, Chan SSM, Wong EKY, Li PYT, et al. History for some or lesson for all? A systematic review and meta-analysis on the immediate and long-term mental health impact of the 2002–2003 severe acute respiratory syndrome (SARS) outbreak. BMC Public Health 2021;21:670. https://doi.org/10.1186/s12889-021-10701-3.

[16] Fowler JC, Cope N, Knights J, Fang H, Skubiak T, Shergill SS, et al. Hummingbird study: results from an exploratory trial assessing the performance and acceptance of a digital medicine system in adults with schizophrenia, schizoaffective disorder, or first-episode psychosis. Neuropsychiatr Dis Treat 2021;17:483–92. https://doi.org/10.2147/NDT.S290793.

[17] Hong JS, Sheriff R, Smith K, Tomlison A, Saad F, Smith T, et al. Impact of COVID-19 on telepsychiatry at the service and individual patient level across two UK NHS mental health trusts. Evid Based Ment Health 2021;24:161–6. https://doi.org/10.1136/ebmental-2021-300287.

[18] Bakolis I, Stewart R, Baldwin D, Beenstock J, Bibby P, Broadbent M, et al. Changes in daily mental health service use and mortality at the commencement and lifting of COVID-19 'lockdown' policy in 10 UK sites: a regression discontinuity in time design. BMJ Open 2021;11, e049721. https://doi.org/10.1136/bmjopen-2021-049721.

[19] Department of Health. Best research for best health - a new national health research strategy. London: Department of Health; 2006.

[20] Delanerolle G, Zeng Y, Shi JQ, Yeng X, Goodison W, Shetty A, Shetty S, Haque N, Elliot K, Ranaweera S, Ramakrishnan R, Raymont V, Rathod S, Phiri P. Mental health impact of the Middle East respiratory syndrome, SARS, and COVID-19: a comparative systematic review and meta-analysis. World J Psychiatry 2022;12(5):739–65. https://doi.org/10.5498/wjp.v12.i5.739.

5

Primary and secondary care research

Key messages

- Within the United Kingdom, clinical research takes place primarily within primary and secondary care services.

- Evidence-based medicine is key factor to improve the designing and delivering primary and secondary care research.

- Evidence-based decision-making means a difference between primary and secondary care should be anticipated.

- Primary and secondary care research should develop specific frameworks that are easily followed by industry and non-commercial entities wanting to deliver research studies in the United Kingdom.

- Funding allocations should be efficiently used to develop research delivery pathways across primary and secondary care organisations in the UK.

5.1 Introduction [1–11]

The Cochrane report in 1972 demonstrated the need to improve quality that is driven by evidence within the National Health Service (NHS). The evidence generated should be driven by way of robust scientific studies using epidemiological and clinical trial methods. Cochrane's approach continues to support evidence-based-medicine (EBM) using retrospective and prospective data. The complexities of data and their constructs are required at two different facets in the United Kingdom, which constitutes primary and secondary care services. The notions of quality of care and exploration of contemporary ideas and innovative methods to improve clinical practice and policies should be reviewed in a patient-centric manner.

The structure of EBM is driven by interrelated constructs of society, individual, healthcare community, and healthcare system (Fig. 5.1). Society represents epidemiologists characterised by

Clinical Trials and Tribulations. https://doi.org/10.1016/B978-0-12-821787-0.00003-9

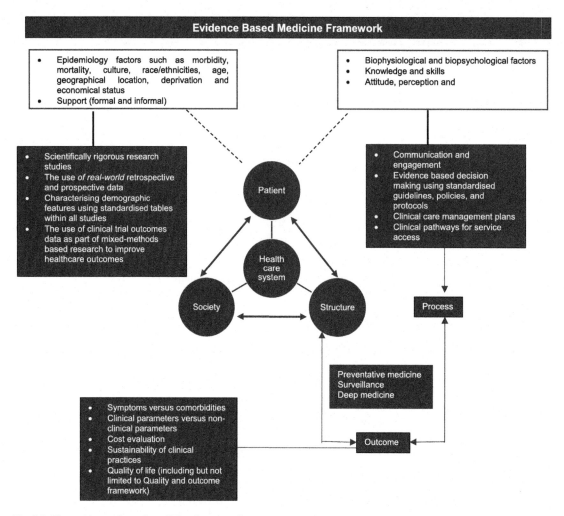

Fig. 5.1 The evidence-based medicine framework.

variables such as socioeconomic status, employment, morbidity, and mortality. The cultural component comprises of an anthropological framework, whilst community resembles professional, formal, and informal networks. Knowledge connects these constructs along with skills, biopsychological components such as attitudes, health beliefs, and perceptions by way of processes. Process quality is dependent on evidence-based decision-making, communication, and clinical management. The development of protocols, guidelines, and algorithms to underpin structured processes is the most effective approach to use for efficient continuous interactions.

Patient-reported outcomes

Patient-reported outcomes (PROs) are based on the outcomes of communication and engagement between doctors and patients. The perception of a shift in the disease outcomes is part of the problem-oriented or goal-oriented outlooks and would equally be part of PROs. A simple example in such a situation would be management of asthma. Minimising of asthma exacerbation events is an important composite of clinical management. This consideration includes optimal symptom management, physical function, and overall quality of life of the patient which is part of patient satisfaction and social equity. The complexities around these components in relation to care offered and definition of quality could be mechanistic and part of EBM.

Medical evidence

Medical evidence has increased over many decades although core clinical questions and gaps in clinical evidence are still present. Depending on the clinical questions, various scientific methodological approaches would be used to critically appraise the data to obtain outcomes. EBM relies on both epidemiology and clinical trial data to have been obtained from well-defined settings of primary and secondary healthcare services. Primary care may also be referred to as 'family practice' and/or 'general practice' in some parts of the world [12]. Often there could be issues between clinical practice and clinical research defining illnesses and representation across age, gender, ethnicities, presence, or absence of comorbidities and social demographic status. The non-specificity of symptoms in some diseases and evolving communicable diseases that lack a generalised diagnosis adds to this complexity. This is further complicated by multimorbidity patients in whom two or more diseases have been diagnosed which subsequently leads to polypharmacy. Thus, the hierarchy of evidence is vital to understand.

5.2 Evidence synthesis

Synthesising evidence is a process that gathers data from a variety of sources and disciplines to inform clinical questions. The decision-making process associated with evidence synthesis is vital for a multitude of stakeholders including policy-makers, clinicians, clinical researchers, patients, and the general public.

The task of making sense of differing sets of data on a given topic was relatively easy in the early decades of science, for the obvious reason that databases, as well as theoretical references, were small. At present, evidence syntheses could be deemed complex and time-consuming although there are many novel methods used. High-quality evidence syntheses would be based on a robust systematic methodology. However, often the inclination has been to define evidence synthesis with systematic reviews, as historically researchers made a conscious effort to conduct singular techniques to report on gathered evidence. Evidence synthesis is also a core component of evidence-based medicine (EBM) which is an explicit, judicious, and modern scientific method to report on evidence to improve the decision-making process, also referred to as evidence-based decisions (EBD). EBM and EBD collectively would be considered as evidence-based healthcare (EBH) which combines the conceptual and practical approaches at a population level. Hence, EBH outcomes are commonly associated with epidemiology research. Indubitably, EBH links clinical research and clinical practice.

The conceptual and policy-level evidence is generated from all the levels demonstrated in Fig. 5.2. However, at present, systematic reviews and meta-analysis generate the most robust scientific outcomes.

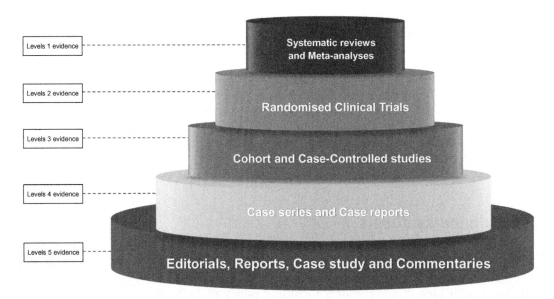

Fig. 5.2 A hierarchical pyramid of scientific evidence. Each level corresponds to the robustness of the scientific methods and the quality of the resulting outcomes. The levels of clinical research emphasise the principles of EBM which drive EBD and EBH where the transition of each step is based on scientific evidence from clinical research and clinical experience.

Systematic review and meta-analyses [13]

A systematic review (SR) can be defined as a structured and rigorous review of evidence to answer a clear research question. SRs use structured methods to identify, select, and critically evaluate relevant data from existing peer-reviewed publications. The premise of extracting this data to conduct a suitable pooled analysis is an attractive feature of an SR. Not all SRs will have meta-analyses since it is an analytical method. Traditionally, SRs have been completed using quantitative approaches within a specific objective. The comprehensiveness of the search process is key to ensuring that the findings are meaningful, scientifically justifiable, and a true representation of the research. Mixed-methods SRs are becoming more popular where both quantitative and qualitative studies are included within the investigation. This also means there are a number of data synthesis and analysis methods that are used to report SRs.

The [14,15] main characteristics that differentiate SR from any other evidence synthesis method is the specificity, transparency, and replicability [16] of the findings that allow a summary of all the data published within a particular context. The systematic search process, for example, is an objective way to pool data-reducing biases. SRs can also use qualitative and quantitative data alongside grey literature, enabling a more comprehensive way to answer a research question. This could lead to the development of new theories and reporting clinical implications that impact policy, clinical practice, and future research.

Designing [17] a suitable methodology is another important facet of an SR. Using the *Population, Intervention, Comparator, and Outcome* (PICO) method is a robust way to ensure the key components are considered to develop an SR protocol as shown in Table 5.1. Alternative methods that could be used include *Sample, Phenomenon of interest, Design, Evaluation, and Research type* (SPIDER) and *Population, Intervention, Comparator, Outcome, and Study type* (PICOS) which can be used within the correct scope. A structured conceptual framework is an important component to develop an SR protocol that demonstrates the rationale, hypothesis, and methods intended to be used to formulate the synthesis of the data. The protocol would also define the use of a meta-analysis, where applicable.

Two examples of developing research questions using suitable PICOs for SRs are shown in Table 5.2.

Key steps to publish a high-quality SR is shown below:
Step 1: Develop a research question
As with any type of research study, developing a robust research question is important as the overall aims and outcomes

Table 5.1 Details relating to the PICO method which can be used to develop a systematic review protocol.

Population	Intervention or exposure	Comparison or control	Outcome
Population characteristics that are required to answer the research question should be affirmed alongside of the clinical condition.	The intervention provided to the population should be selected. Selecting a single or multiple exposures at the onset of the SR is important to be considered for the purpose of developing a eligibility criteria.	A comparison or control population aligned to the intervention or exposures would be useful. However, some research questions may not require a control or comparison within the context of an SR.	Common outcomes reported in SRs include morbidity, mortality, adverse events, etc.

Table 5.2 Two examples of how research questions can be developed using the PICO method.

Research question	Population	Intervention or exposure	Comparison or control	Outcome
What is the prevalence of hypertension among patients with chronic kidney disease?	Patients with hypertension and chronic kidney disease of all genders above the age of 18 years of age	Exposure is chronic kidney disease patients diagnosed with hypertension	No comparison or control	Potential outcomes include morbidity, complications and rates of complications
What is the rate of use of analgesics among amputees suffering from phantom limb pain?	Patient with phantom limb pain that have had amputations	Interventions are Analgesics such as Gabapentin, Morphine and Codeine.	Compare each intervention listed across all genders and age groups. A control group can also be included where patients who are not taking any analgesics for the condition.	Potential outcomes include decreased pain symptoms, morbidity, and complications

will need to be aligned to be reported within this scope. A good method to develop a research question would be to keep the PICO method (Population, Intervention, Comparator, and Outcome) in mind. A *reverse engineered* approach could be used.

Step 2: Systematic review protocol

An SR protocol details the research question, aims, objectives, eligibility criteria, methods used to gather and analyse data. SR protocols should be published as part of good practice. The International Prospective Register of Systematic Reviews (PROSPERO) is a good place to register an SR although there are many journals that publish that could be used. The transparent reporting of systematic reviews and meta-analyses (PRISMA) guidelines should be used as part of developing the protocol.

Step 3: Developing a search strategy

The first step with developing a search strategy is establishing keywords that could be used along with established Medical Subject Headings (MeSH) aligned to the research question and PICO. MeSH is a comprehensive vocabulary thesaurus that indexes peer-reviewed publications for PubMed. MeSH vocabulary comprises four main types of terms of subheadings, headings, concept records, and features of the publication. Search engines such as ScienceDirect have their own database of MeSH terms and keywords that can be used. Ovid, EBSCO, CINAHL, and MEDLINE are other platforms that could be used. Study registers could also be included as part of the search strategy, such as ClinicalTrials. gov, Drugs@FDA, and ISRCTN. The regulatory database, Drugs@FDA is particularly useful for SRs assessing side effects of drugs or medical devices.

Once the search engines provide an output, study titles and abstracts should be reviewed. Most search engines have an option to exclude duplicates as well as publications that are not research studies. The full set of articles can then be downloaded into the worksheet that has been prepared for the study. Alternatively, SR software such as EndNote can be used to review the full-text articles.

Steps 1–4 should be used to develop a suitable data extraction template as below using excel and/or a statistical software as *R* or ANOVA (Fig. 5.3).

Step 5: Data extraction

The data extraction step has four mini-steps and is as follows:

- Each included study should have a full paper available to review the abstract first to ensure the eligibility criteria has been met.
- Each paper should be further reviewed using the full content.
- The data extraction should commence in line with the data constructed template.
- Data extraction sheet should be checked and verified by two independent reviewers.

	A	B	C	D	E	F	G	H	I	J	K
1	Study long title	Journal	Author	Objectives	Other Findings	Study Type	Symptoms	Sample Size	Publication Year	Study Period (Start - End)	Country
2											
3											

	L	M	N	O	P	Q	R	S	T	U	V
1	Setting	Inclusion/Exclusion Criteria	Mean age	Exposure	Outcome	Outcome code	Outcome assessment	Prevalence	Median	IQR	Range
2											
3											

	W	X	Y	Z	AA	AB	AC	AD	AE
1	Mean	SD	Mean difference	Odds ratio	Relative risk	Hazard ratio	Confidence interval	p-value	References identified
2									
3									

Fig. 5.3 An example of a data extraction template in Excel.

This type of extraction sheet allows a researcher to synthesise the evidence and make any adjustments to the analysis plan including a meta-analysis.

Step 6: Analyses

Once the data set for the analysis has been completed, the effect size should be assessed. This step aids with deciding to complete a statistical synthesis and/or a meta-analyses. The data extraction sheet can be used to assess the type of result tables to generate in relation to the analyses. A comprehensive SR analysis can be a combination of a narrative synthesis and a descriptive analysis. These can be tabulated in addition to conducting a risk of bias and sensitivity assessment. A PRISMA checklist and PRISMA diagram should be completed. SR and meta-analyses are a vital for evidence synthesis and should be completed prior to conducting a clinical trial or an epidemiology study to identify research gaps that require addressing. This is an important facet for EBM and improving clinical practices.

Personalised medicine

Personalised medicine is defined as individualised clinical care to treat diseases. The use of this method aims at optimising the efficacy and effectiveness of patient care whilst also reducing costs. Drugs and medical device manufacturers would equally benefit from personalised medicine. The World Health Organisation (WHO) and The International Consortium for Personalised

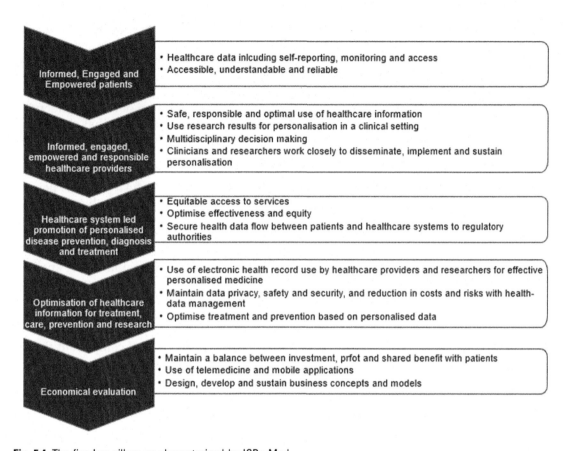

Fig. 5.4 The five key pillars as characterised by ICPerMed.

Medicine (ICPerMed) support the advancement of the biomedical, socioeconomic, and technological driving forces to promote research innovations prior to implementation within clinical practice. ICPerMed characterised five key pillars that should be implemented by 2030 to improve diagnostics, treatments, and prevention (Fig. 5.4).

Primary care research

Primary care research in the United Kingdom is a rewarding yet challenging enterprise given that approximately 80% of clinical consultations take place. Historically, conducting primary care research has been a low priority for clinicians in the United Kingdom as general practices have been independent, and the ethos has been clinical care for patients being a priority. This has changed over the last two decades where there has been growth of resources by way of the development of the UK clinical research network (UK-CRN) for primary care and relationships between clinical academics, services, providers and general practitioners. The CRN has supported primary care secure infrastructure necessary to conduct research although the divulge nations of England, Scotland, Wales, and Northern Ireland have developed independent approaches to deliver the required work. This has also meant that challenges associated within primary care tend to be more diverse for an increasing population.

A fraction of primary care healthcare professionals are involved with academic centres and/or industry to take part in acute medicine research studies. There are possible historical reasons for this where biomedical research has centred on acute care and/or basic sciences where mechanistic evolvement of diseases is considered the central focus despite the diagnostic pathways all diseases starting within primary care. Clinical inertia is another facet alongside implementation delays associated with any discoveries developed. Research has also felt more of a professional responsibility underpinned by moral and ethical implications associated with medicine; thus, practitioner involvement varies.

Community and primary care are another component that is important to develop and conduct high-quality research, especially for communicable diseases and the advancement of digital [18] technologies. The use of primary care healthcare records, for example, is a rich source to develop better clinical tools. For example, the use of primary care data from the Clinical Practice Research Datalink (CPRD) has assisted psychiatrists to better evaluate mental-health-related prescribing practices within the United Kingdom where the data linkage has enabled policy-makers to evaluate safety and long-term implications of anti-psychotic drug use. This type of research allowed policy-makers to also consider better cost-effective models to be used when commissioning groups consider primary care practice payments. In addition, inadequate medication monitoring and key indicating to determine inter-practice variation could also be considered within primary care.

Evolving primary and secondary care services could assist with advancing communicable and emergency-medicine-based research. The establishment of walk-in-centres (WICs) was a good opportunity to manage the rise in emergency department attendance which has been challenging for most hospitals within the United Kingdom. A more multidisciplinary approach also means efforts to better manage patients that require urgent care services which would be beneficial to the general public and for healthcare services in the long term to develop novel services, such as those led by allied healthcare professionals. For example, nurse-practitioners-led WICs were established to improve minor illness and injury management 7 days a week where GPs are also available. It was reported that patients were more satisfied in comparison to GP practices due to a number of reasons including easy access and shorter waiting times [19]. However, the continuity of care and safety implications have been raised by GPs and some patients which led to the establishment of GP-led WICs aimed to reduce emergency department admissions. However, the models of care between these WICs were similar. These centres were not involved with research despite the importance of exploring these routinely gathered data in conjunction with primary and acute healthcare research studies.

Clinical trials of drugs and medical devices in primary care are another aspect that has not grown as much as hospital-based work, despite having good opportunities to recruit a more diverse array of patients. Most clinical trials within primary care focus on complex interventions and/or educational programs. These are important aspects, although the clinical impact can be less in comparison to that of testing a drug or medical device. The importance of primary care practice-based recruitment has been demonstrated during the COVID-19 pandemic. Similar, if not the same, recruitment enrichment strategies could be introduced to clinical trials that have historically focused in larger hospitals. A split-recruitment approach could also assist with meeting recruitment targets and potentially increase sample sizes, especially for rare diseases. This would be relatively straightforward for larger GP practices with the presence of pharmacists and/or nurse practitioners. GP practices also have the potential to act as a participant identification centre in order to be part of drug or medical device trials.

Secondary care research

Within the United Kingdom, all acute medicine specialties are part of secondary care organisations, and majority of these conduct many different types of secondary care research. The COVID-19 pandemic demonstrated the link between clinical research and better outcomes, as well as the ability of the NHS to deliver research remotely. Whilst there are challenges around resourcing drug and medical device trials, sustaining an adaptable research ecosystem across 80+ hospitals can be cumbersome, especially since research extends beyond the scope of novel medicine approaches. Acceleration of study setup and delivery for communicable and non-communicable diseases are important.

This is dependent on a number of factors including resources, governance approvals, and contractual agreements.

Acute medicine specialties are key to providing specialist care to patients, thus any research conducted within these organisations provides useful data to better understand clinical problems.

Case study

Assessing disease sequalae is an important component of clinical practice. This is a complex area of medicine to diagnose, treat, and manage. Therefore, gathering evidence as efficiently as possible to either demonstrate limited evidence availability which is rate limiting for clinical management or issues with clinical management that could lead to multimorbidity is helpful for clinicians and researchers to understand to develop better ways to support patients. An important first step could be to conduct an SR and meta-analyses to assess disease sequalae. This is a relatively new scientific method to better identify and report research evidence to inform clinical practice. This is also a good method to assess emerging evidence that could systematically synthesise symptoms.

Learning objectives

Conducting a comprehensive SR and meta-analysis exploring disease sequalae that is aligned to the research question with clear outcomes requires the completion of all necessary steps although completing a robust data extraction method is key. A few other learning objectives are listed below:

- An effective disease sequalae could be established by extracting the data using an '*adaptive*' data collection method. Before commencing the extraction, a suitable template should be designed covering all potential statistical and non-statistical composites of the identified study.
- Mixed-methods approaches can be used to report SR and meta-analyses that can be useful to explore bidirectionality of a complex clinical problem.
- The data extraction should be checked and verified by an independent reviewer ideally prior to starting the analyses.
- To maximise the use of the data gathered, clear statistical methods should be considered. A planned statistical analysis plan is useful to have at the beginning of the study although these methods should amend if the data gathered show further analytical methods are required.
- Qualitative studies can be used within SRs and meta-analyses. Before using this information, researchers should decide if they wish to include this as part of a descriptive analysis and/or quantitative analyses. Qualitative data can be

transformed into a statistical assimilation. Nominal and ordinal scales can be used to measure qualitative data.

- Computer software programs are available to manage qualitative and quantitative data when completing a meta-analysis.
- Mixed methods could provide pattern recognition to show regularities or peculiarities that could characterise the data in a structured way for reporting purposes. This would allow distinctions to be drawn between the primary and secondary condition, vice versa.

References

[1] Hobbs R. Is primary care research important and relevant to GPs? Br J Gen Pract 2019;69(686):424–5. https://doi.org/10.3399/bjgp19X705149.

[2] Adams PF, Benson V. Current estimates from the National Health Interview Survey, 1991. Vital Health Stat 1992;184:1–232.

[3] Barondess JA. Content and process in ambulatory care. Am J Med 1982;73:735–9. https://doi.org/10.1016/0002-9343(82)90417-x.

[4] Blackhall LJ, Murphy ST, Frank G, Michel V, Azen S. Ethnicity and attitudes toward patient autonomy. JAMA 1995;274:820–5.

[5] Carrese JA, Rhodes LA. Western bioethics on the Navajo reservation: benefit or harm? JAMA 1995;274:826–9.

[6] Evidence-Based Medicine Working Group. Evidence-based medicine: a new approach to teaching the practice of medicine. JAMA 1992;268:2420–5. https://doi.org/10.1001/jama.1992.03490170092032.

[7] Hofmans-Okkes I, Lamberts H. Episodes of care and the large majority of personal health care needs: is the new IOM definition of primary care reflected in U.S. primary care data? Paper commissioned by the Institute of Medicine Committee on the Future of Primary Care; 1995.

[8] Kasper JF, Mulley AG, Wennberg JE. Developing shared decision-making programs to improve the quality of health care. Qual Rev Bull 1992;18:183–90. https://doi.org/10.1016/s0097-5990(16)30531-0.

[9] Klinkman MS, Green LA. Using ICPC in a computer-based primary care information system. Fam Med 1995;27:449–56.

[10] Lalonde M. A new perspective on the health of Canadians. Ottawa: Ministry of National Health and Welfare; 1974.

[11] Lamberts H, Hofmans-Okkes I. Characteristics of primary care. Episode of care: a core concept in family practice. J Fam Practice 1996;42:161–7.

[12] Szajewska H. Evidence-based medicine and clinical research: both are needed, neither is perfect. Ann Nutr Metab 2018;72(Suppl 3):13–23. https://doi.org/10.1159/000487375.

[13] Page MJ, Moher D, Bossuyt PM, Boutron I, Hoffmann TC, Mulrow CD, et al. PRISMA 2020 explanation and elaboration: updated guidance and exemplars for reporting systematic reviews. BMJ 2021;372, n160. https://doi.org/10.1136/bmj.n160.

[14] Undertaking Systematic Reviews of Research on Effectiveness. CRD's guidance for those carrying out or commissioning reviews. CRD Report Number 4, 2nd Edition. NHS Centre for Reviews and Dissemination, University of York; 2001.

[15] Cochrane Collab. Glossary. London: Rep., Cochrane Collab; 2003. Retrieved from: http://community.cochrane.org/glossary.

[16] Siddaway AP, Wood AM, Hedges LV. How to do a systematic review: a best practice guide for conducting and reporting narrative reviews, meta-analyses, and meta-syntheses. Annu Rev Psychol 2019;4(70):747–70. https://doi.org/10.1146/annurev-psych-010418-102803.

[17] Methley AM, Campbell S, Chew-Graham C, McNally R, Cheraghi-Sohi S. PICO, PICOS and SPIDER: a comparison study of specificity and sensitivity in three search tools for qualitative systematic reviews. BMC Health Serv Res 2014;14:579. https://doi.org/10.1186/s12913-014-0579-0.

[18] Khawagi WY, Steinke D, Carr MJ, Wright AK, Ashcroft DM, Avery A, et al. Evaluating the safety of mental health-related prescribing in UK primary care: a cross-sectional study using the clinical practice research datalink (CPRD). BMJ Qual Safety 2021. https://doi.org/10.1136/bmjqs-2021-013427.

[19] Salisbury C, Manku-Cott T, Moore L, Chalder M, Sharp D. Questionnaire survey of users of NHS walk-in centres: observational study. Br J Gen Pract 2002;52:554–60.

Further reading

Mayer N, Meza-Torres B, Okusi C, Delanerolle G, Chapman M, Wang W, Anand S, Feher M, Macartney J, Byford R, Joy M, Gatenby P, Curcin V, Greenhalgh T, Delaney B, de Lusignan S. Developing a long COVID phenotype for post-acute COVID-19 in a national primary care sentinel cohort: protocol for an observational retrospective database analysis. JMIR Public Health Surveill 2022;8, 36989.

6

Data science and clinical informatics

Key messages

- Data science is an important facet of clinical research.
- Real-world data are useful to improve healthcare outcomes.
- Collating, processing, and analysing data should be aligned to the protocol specific objectives and outcome measures.
- Clinical informatics used to improve healthcare outcomes is becoming more popular.
- Using real-world and clinical trial data in healthcare technology development in the United Kingdom is fit for purpose in comparison to interventions developed in other countries.

6.1   Introduction

Data science aims to provide actionable information based on the vast amount of information available. The real-world data are often unstructured and noisy. The ability to gain insights and make sense of this can provide actionable intel to solve problems. Such an analysis can find new correlations. Considering that few exabytes (2^{60} bytes) of data are generated every day, it is a technical change to store, process, and analyse this. It is beyond the processing power of the traditional software to cope with this as a unification of statistics, data analysis informatics, and machine learning is required. The complex field of realising this objective is data science. This application involves the complex intertwining of other domains such as big data with data mining and artificial intelligence. The data scientist needs to have the domain knowledge in the field of its application to enable him to write programming codes if he were to gain insights from the data.

The digitisation of the healthcare system has resulted in an avalanche of new clinical big data and, consequently, has led to a rapid growth of data science in medicine. Provost and Fawcett,

Clinical Trials and Tribulations. https://doi.org/10.1016/B978-0-12-821787-0.00012-X

in 2013, defined data science as 'the set of fundamental principles that support and guide the extraction of information and knowledge from data' [1]. Therefore, data science is the area of study dedicated to the principle-based extraction of knowledge from broader and more complex data and which has been particularly used in the intensive care setting [2] (Fig. 6.1).

Data science has become the new fuel for companies and is now an integral part of every decision-making process. As the adoption of analytics methods such as data science and big data analytics has increased, so have the challenges in data science. The biggest problems to be faced today have been: (1) data preparation – data scientists spend nearly 80% of their time cleaning and preparing data to improve its quality, i.e. make it accurate and consistent, before using it for analysis; (2) multiple data sources – this process requires manual input of data, which leads to errors and repetitions and, eventually, to bad decisions; and (3) data security – cyber-attacks have become increasingly common, creating a risk to data security [3].

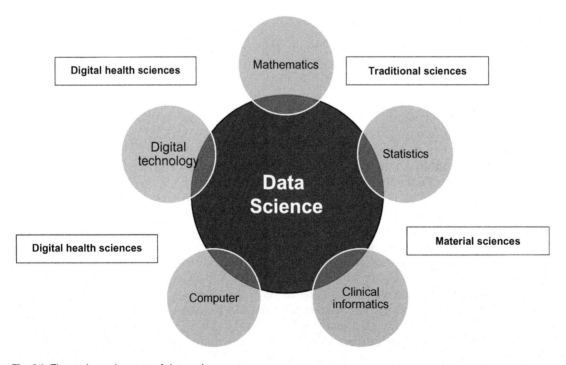

Fig. 6.1 The various elements of data science.

Data and knowledge engineering

Since the 4th Industrial Revolution, also called Revolution 4.0 by some sources, the world has been forced, once and for all, to embark on a technological evolution, which in turn has triggered a continual process of transition. However, even though this technological evolution has significantly improved the health area, such as the standardisation of data extraction, little knowledge has been obtained in this process [4].

Since the introduction of computers to society in the mid-1980s, the medical community (specialising in health management) has rigorously digitised medical activities [5]. However, there is still a fraction of the economically disadvantaged population that still suffers from lack of access to technology [6]. Big data has given medicine a new look today regarding evidence-based knowledge and practice.

Understanding socioeconomic and health disparities is not a simple task. The advancements of big data have been crucial in the organisation of information aimed at facilitating such task by creating a favourable technological environment for this; for example, by increasing access to health through multimodal, multifactorial, and multilevel sources for data mining [4]. Also, by standardising demographic and social information in electronic records [7], improving public health surveillance through the standardisation of demographic information [8], and last but not least, by improving understanding of the aetiology of health disparities and of minority health through modelling and data science. These are examples of the great advantages of data science in healthcare.

Knowledge processing

Knowledge processing has been an integral part of knowledge engineering since the early 1980s [9]. Knowledge engineering concepts are widespread and well accepted in areas such as artificial intelligence [3], specialised systems [4], recognition of standards [5], computer vision [6,7], and even robotics. Accuracy and knowledge are critical to the overall success of a data analysis project. Knowledge can often help us achieve the level accuracy expected. For example, if we want to build a recommendation system for an e-commerce platform, we need to understand how users navigate online stores [10].

In data science, the term domain knowledge is used to refer to general knowledge of the field or environment to which data science methods are being applied. Data science can be defined as the study of tools used to model and/or interpret data, generate insights from data, and make decisions based on data [11].

Currently, data science is being applied in many industry, university, and government organisations, often by self-taught professionals. There is evidence of strong demand in several domains for graduates with data science skills [12]. A study by IBM found more than 2.3 million job offers in science and data analytics in 2015, and openings are expected to grow significantly in the coming years [13,14]. Today's data science programmes are highly variable, can be complex and language-specific. Complex because, in part, emerging educational approaches stem from different institutional contexts, aim to reach students in different communities, address different challenges, and seek to achieve different goals. Data scientists have great potential to help address critical real-world challenges, such as by enabling a more accurate diagnosis of melanomas through better image analysis [15]; improving decision-making [16]; and developing smart cities. In the latter case, data can be processed, analysed, and used to improve the efficiency and cost-effectiveness of cities as well as the well-being of residents [17].

6.2 Clinical informatics [18–24]

Clinical informatics is defined as data captured and communicated knowledge from healthcare professionals and patients, as well as their practices. Informatics in medicine originated in the early 19th century with the use of a data processing systems in the United States which was used for public health surveys that reported population epidemiology outcomes. The basic concepts of clinical informatics are useful to understand its' use and development for future information technology infrastructure in healthcare systems. Information technology systems are built to retain and reuse data as a core entity to verify, report, and analyse patient medical histories. However, by the early 1990s, their use in clinical research became apparent.

Historically, clinical informatics was used for quality improvement projects in acute care and became more popular in applied primary care research, as well as life-course epidemiology. Electronic healthcare record (EHR) systems and electronic data systems (EDCs) can be considered as part of health and clinical informatics research, where both clinical and research data can be used within the scope of the research being explored. The most effective use of data could be a combination of clinical and research data where the unification could promote the enrichment of the

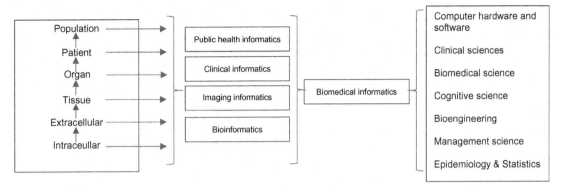

Fig. 6.2 Clinical informatics.

sample and data quality. This work could be used to enhance workflows and information sources to facilitate quality improvements, research capabilities, and processes facilitating high-quality *real-world* research studies (Fig. 6.2).

The combination of clinical informatics and data has untapped powers especially within the NHS. Data within the NHS are rich source clinical information despite variations in data constructs and missing data. Combining general practice (GP) and hospital data could further the value of data sets providing insightful medical histories for tens of millions of patients. Data-driven clinical research has been unfathomable in managing the COVID-19 pandemic with diverse data sets that could aid in refining clinical care and ongoing management. To achieve effective use of clinical informatics, coding nomenclature used across all healthcare services and their accurate mapping to clinical terminologies should be affirmed.

Medicine is intrinsically complex and therefore inherently challenging to design and develop fit-for-purpose clinical informatic systems that are easily adaptable to the demands over short, medium, and long term. Health data in the United Kingdom like many healthcare systems have incompatible formats, making the data harvesting process to become inconsistent. Classification informatic systems could be useful to develop semi-automated integration and linkage with different data sets to general web-ontology language (OWL). OWL describes the terms of properties, classes, and individual descriptions of characteristics. OWL can be used to develop tools and ontologies in various clinical and scientific areas that were not compatible with the semantic web. These have been further developed by way of computational notation and integrating temporal semantics to use as an eligibility checker for clinical trials.

6.3 Interoperability [25–27]

Interoperability in health and social care has various definitions and is complex in nature. The ability to formulate information systems, applications, devices, and their integration in a coordinated manner at multiple levels in a seamless manner allows clinical informatics use in clinical research. Standardised nomenclature requires common definitions to enable interoperability between healthcare systems that could be categorised as technical, semantic, and process interoperability where there is a lack of interoperability within EHRs in the United Kingdom. Within the United Kingdom, HER interoperability concerns are emphasised due to the adoption of primary and secondary medical care records for the purpose of real-world research to improve clinical and patient-reported outcomes [28]. Several quality improvement projects in the United Kingdom have highlighted that the lack of parity also impacts evidence-based decision-making (EBD), which impacts clinical practice. Large-scale integration within the NHS is another concern; therefore, exploring the three categories would be important for any researcher attempting to use informatics methods in clinical research.

Technical interoperability

Technical interoperability is defined as a process that moved data between systems across multiple layers. The architecture of the data construct and exchange, inferences to application, and standardisation of these require secure servers, as well as a robust understanding of clinical area being explored and the technical components required to process the data. This could be categorised under multiple levels as shown below:

- Level 1 is considered as the foundation level associated with establishing the inter-connectivity requirements for the system required to transfer and receive the data
- Level 2 is defined as the syntax and format of the data filed required for interpretation
- Level 3 is referred to as the semantic level where common data models and unified coding or coding mapping techniques are used to standardised the definitions. This is also the step where the digital and clinical phenotypes are brought to life.
- Level 4 is considered as the research governance, legal and policy considerations required to facilitate the use of the data associated with the research study. This component uses an integrated approach by combining end-user processes and workflows to use the data in an efficient and effective manner.

Semantic interoperability

Semantic interoperability consists of data exchange from the recipient's perspective. These coded terminologies and messaging schemes are used to exchange information between NHS organisations using semantic technologies. The next generation of Web has been called the semantic web. The semantic web is an extension of the current web, whose main function is to provide information not only to humans, but also to help machines understand and interpret data. Berners-Lee et al. believe that this form of web content is useful for computers to spark a revolution of new possibilities [29]. The term semantic technologies represent a range of technologies that have been around for a long time and seek to help derive meaning from information. Some examples of semantic technologies include: natural language processing (NLP), data mining, artificial intelligence (AI), category tagging, and semantic search [30].

Process evaluation

Process evaluation associated with clinical informatics focuses on process interoperability where the integrations of systems within workflow process are used to build an 'informatics ecosystem'. Obstacles to this form of interoperability include heterogeneous data, complexity associated with clinical knowledge, and lack of standardisation, as well as misunderstanding between end users and systems. Process evaluations are in general twofold, when clinical informatics are in use in the context of clinical research.

6.4 Electronic health records (EHRs)

In the United Kingdom, there are different EHRs used between primary, secondary, and tertiary healthcare organisations [31], in addition to intra-institutional variations with the NHS. Leveraging existing data from these systems then requires the development of standard terminologies and ontologies that are digitally and clinically relevant. Digital phenotypes could be translated to clinical phenotypes, and vice versa, if the ontologies developed remain accurate [31]. Therefore, validating these is not challenging. However, curating lists of standardised terminologies can be complicated due to a number of reasons including the difference in nomenclature use between the divulged nations in the United Kingdom. Thus, ICD 10, SNOMED CT, Readv2, and dm + dx are used across various networks. Whilst there have been attempts to develop common data models [32], there have been challenges around the unification of codes. As a result, mapping protocols at present appear to be a more effective albeit time-consuming.

Another similar approach is the use of performance of term-binding algorithms for SNOMED CT terms and Archetype elements where the terms could use term alignment. A working example of this that was successfully implemented was with the human genome project. Apart from SNOMED CT, Read codes and ICD10 are used within healthcare services in the United Kingdom. England, Scotland, Wales, and Northern Ireland use SNOMED CT, Read, and ICD10 codes respectively in primary care services whilst secondary care uses ICD10 and ICD9, where applicable. An important difference in the method of coding within primary and secondary care services is the involvement of clinicians and coding specialists, respectively. The number of new terms also grows, and thereby the previously implemented simple hierarchical structures and designs have outgrown. Similarly, EHR system designs require changing to befit all other changes to reflect the correct content. The transition of Read to SNOMED CT is another aspect that will deliver further changes to the extraction and use of coded clinical information in research. Table 6.1 demonstrates differences between SNOMED CT and Read along with quality assurance issues.

Data quality issues

It is advised the use of coded data in clinical research should be verified before any analysis is conducted, especially if the sample includes those from divulge nations. Therefore, as a general rule, primary care clinicians and clinical coding teams in hospitals are encouraged to use the code closest to the clinical condition, treatment, and other information. It is encouraged that remaining consistent across patients could reduce potential data quality issues. The following are examples of correctly coding clinical information:

- Use the code for Salmonella gastroenteritis (disorder) if a patient was diagnosed with this condition instead of Salmonella
- Use lymphadenopathy than lymph node which is a body structure
- Use alcohol abuse instead of alcohol

A common recording issue is the use of occupational terms especially within the Read where patient's occupations are recorded in addition to those of the treating healthcare professional. For example, *doctor* is often used instead of *referral to doctor*. Training staff to record information correctly regularly could

Table 6.1 The differences between SNOMED CT and Read along.

Key characteristics	SNOMED CT	Readv2	ICD10	dm+dx	Quality assurance issues
Character length of the code	6–18 digits	5 digits	3–7 digits [33]	4–6 alphanumeric digits	
Type of term	Indicated by hierarchy and fully specified name (FSN)	Indication is inferred from the actual code	To identify adverse drug events, classify and code all diagnoses. [34]	Identify diabetes and whether insulin dependent or not with more complications.	
Parent codes	Multiple codes	1 code	Multiple codes	Multiple codes	A single parental code is not Always representative clinically and could lead to duplicated. Multiple parental codes are more reflective of the clinical context although
Hierarchies	No limitations for depth	A limit of 5 levels in depth			Limitations could prevent effectively and accurately representing a condition
Incorrect codes	Outdated concepts and changes to clinical conditions could be amended, thereby the code	Incorrect terms and codes cannot be removed	Reimbursements to get delayed, denied, or only partially paid. [35]	Not applicable	The likelihood of errors are higher in Read than SNOMED CT.

Continued

Table 6.1 The differences between SNOMED CT and Read along—cont'd

Key characteristics	SNOMED CT	Readv2	ICD10	dm+dx	Quality assurance issues
Discpriptors	Terms such as NOS and NEC (not otherwise specified and not elsewhere classified, respectively) are unavailable	Not applicable	Terms such as NOS and NEC (not otherwise specified and not elsewhere classified, respectively) are unavailable [36].	Diabetes mellitus due to underlying condition without complications. E08. 9 is a billable/specific ICD-10-CM code that can be used to indicate a diagnosis for reimbursement purposes. The 2022 edition of ICD-10-CM E08 [37].	Reducing ambiguity is based on the use of correct clinical concepts which is an important principle of SNOMED CT. Each concept comprises of descriptions that define the concept. Some of these are e more precise although at least single unambiguous descriptions could exist. This is not the case for Read. Therefore, if both SNOMED CT and Read codes are used for research studies or within analytical reports, mapping the correct definitions are important.

Table 6.1 The differences between SNOMED CT and Read along—cont'd

Key characteristics	SNOMED CT	Readv2	ICD10	dm+dx	Quality assurance issues
Abbreviated terms	Abbreviated terms in Read are not used in SNOMEDCT		During code searchers, abbreviated forms of words could be used.		During code searchers, abbreviated forms of words could be used.
Duplicate terms	A single concept ID is used therefore lacks duplication	Duplicate terms in Read have been grouped to a single concept in SNOMED CT	Errors can be fixed during the filling.		Spelling errors should be corrected and any outdated terms need to be removed manually.
Synonyms	True synonyms	Similar synonyms		Similar synonyms	Using Read and SNOMED CT codes in the same context
Code hierarchy for differential diagnosis	Code for NOT this condition are present	Codes for NOT this condition are lacking	Code for differential diagnosis in mental health disorders is available.		

improve data quality issues. To address some of these issues, the following steps could be used:

- Singular instead of plural terms should be used when carrying forth searches
- Spaces should not be used pre or post the use of a hyphen when searches are created. For example, the word *intraarticular* should be written as *intra-articular*
- Apostrophes should be avoided, for example, *Down's Syndrome* should be written as *Down Syndrome*
- Non-significant words such as *of* or *the* should be avoided
- The use of 2–3 words with at least four characters could be used when searches are conducted in systems

- Exploring the descendants and ancestors of SNOMED CT hierarchy would be useful to determine if the correct concept has been finalised

Duplicate terms are another issue surrounding data quality. There are a number of terms in Readv2 that have had issues with duplication either due to the categorization method or an error. This issue has improved in recent years given that there are software used to check, verify, and validate any duplication issues at the authoring stage prior to a release of terms which are formalised. Another facet of this issue would be that such duplicate codes could be mapped to the same SNOMED CT concept with a different description. For example:

- A130. Tuberculous meningitis and F004. Meningitis tuberculous; these are mapped to a single SNOMED CT term of tuberculous meningitis
- F583. 00 Tinnitus 1C2. 00 Tinnitus symptoms F583Z 00 Tinnitus NOS; these are mapped to a single SNOMED CT term 101,130,017 Tinnitus
- 8764. Nebuliser therapy 74,592 Nebuliser therapy; these are mapped to a single SNOMED CT term of Nebuliser therapy

Word order, plural nouns, and spelling errors

SNOMED CT has editorial principles with specific text descriptions, thus more consistent in comparison to Read codes. As such the *word order* of terms could alter and use additional symbols such as hyphens. Examples of these are follows:

- 3712. 00 Naso-lacrimal duct probing maps to 90,246,009 Probing of nasolacrimal duct
- 533.. 00 Soft tissue X-ray neck maps to 168,719,007 Neck soft tissue X-ray

SNOMED CT editing rules recommend avoiding the use of plural nouns where Read does not, which could reflect in the mapping process. For example:

- 01.... 00 Top managers maps to 265,911,003 Top manager
- 1B8.. 00 Eye symptoms maps to 308,923,001 Eye symptom

Any errors observed in Readv2 cannot be corrected if the original text included into the EHR is saved. On the other hand, SNOMED CT has the ability manage this and outdated terms are removed. For example, diabetes mellitus is currently described as type 1 or type 2 than the older version of inclusion or non-insulin-dependent. Older Readv2 terms are not available in SNOMED CT, as shown below:

- C10E. Type 1 diabetes mellitus (version 2) X40J4 Type I diabetes mellitus (CTV3)

- C10F. Type 2 diabetes mellitus (version 2) X40J5 Type II diabetes mellitus (CTV3)
  Instead of;
- C108. Insulin-dependent diabetes mellitus
- C109 Non-insulin-dependent diabetes mellitus
  This would result in a mapping table with the following;
  C10E. 12 Insulin-dependent diabetes mellitus maps to 46,635,009 Type 1 diabetes mellitus.

Mapping read to SNOMED CT codes

For researchers that use coded data, terminology mapping is required. Whilst the UK terminology Centre (UKTC) could be used to map SNOMED CT codes to Read terms, consistency could be an issue due to differing approaches taken by GPs and GP systems that derive equivalent descriptions. Mapping tables have been produced using a combination of automatic technologies and manual mapping methods. Selective manual checking is used as a quality control step. Mapping tables are freely available within UKTC's distribution site referred to as TRUD.

The observational medical outcomes partnership (OMOP) common data model (CDM) is another approach that could be used for standardising vocabularies [32]. However, the use of CDMs could have rate-limiting factors within the United Kingdom. The specifications of the CDM have been agreed by the OHDSI community and the vocabulary is available for download in the Athena web portal (https://athena.ohdsi.org/search-terms/start).

Terms in Readv2 in NOS (not otherwise specified), NES (not elsewhere classified), or HFQ (however further qualified) and those OS (other specified) are based on the ICD classifications. Pre- and post-fixed meanings can be specific and unique although new codes are added every few years. These act as 'catch-alls' that lack a specific code within the relevant classification. Codes can also be added for a condition in downstream versions which would mean there would be lag in capturing valuable clinical information. This is another limitation in Readv2 in comparison to SNOMED CT.

SNOMED CT is updated 6 monthly, thus 'catch-alls' term preservation is minimal. 'Catch-alls' term lacks a well-defined meaning within a terminology that provides the vocabulary used to describe the relevant details in patient records. When mapping Read to SNOMED CT, these terms can be mapped to SNOMED CT synonym without the NOS/NEC/HFQ/Other specified or generic codes. A few examples are shown below:
- F52z. 00 Otitis MEDIA NOS maps to 65,363,002 Otitis media
- Q4z.. 15 Stillbirth NEC maps to 237,364,002 Stillbirth

- 71,244 00 Biopsy of lesion of adrenal gland NEC maps to 172,033,008 Biopsy of lesion of adrenal gland
- 7A5z. 00 Other artery operations NOS maps to 118,805,000 Procedure on artery

Abbreviation length is a considerable limitation in Readv2 in comparison to SNOMED CT which lacks such restrictions to avoid ambiguity. System suppliers such as NHS digital or EMIS accommodate longer descriptions and unabbreviated equivalent terms. Examples of these are below

- 24F8. 00 O/E – L.dorsalis pedis present maps to 163120009 On examination-left dorsalis pedis pulse present
- 124.1 00FH: * – gastrointestinal tract maps to 429006005 Family history of malignant neoplasm of gastrointestinal tract
- 2691. 00 O/E – vaginal speculum exam. NAD maps to 163413007 On examination – vaginal speculum examination – not abnormality detected

Common clinical abbreviations exist in SNOMED CT which is a synonym, and the full explanation of the abbreviation will appear within the same descriptor. For example, a synonym is unavailable for COPD – chronic obstructive pulmonary disease. This is due to differences in meanings among varying specialties. For example, PID may mean **pelvic inflammatory disease** or **prolapsed intervertebral disc**. SNOMED comprises a more conservation abbreviation list for treatment to ensure misinterpretation if shared within another HER.

Data variable curation

Clinical data curation is highly complex and often unappreciated within the scientific community mostly due to the lack of understanding and knowledge available to describe specificity within codes. There are limitations to data curation although it is applied to all patient records. Some patient records have more than one clinical code and could often cause contradictions and even misunderstandings when analytical methods are used. This is a common issue when coded information is used in research studies. The nature of the codes is as such, developing a digital phenotype and suitable ontology could be useful to interpret findings using coding classifications. For example, coding schema and the relative missingness vary across different electronic systems, especially within primary care as demonstrated in Table 6.2.

The medicines dictionary used in the United Kingdom; British National Formulary (BNF) comprises information on all medicines, dressing, and appliances prescribed in the United Kingdom along with information on side effects and doses. There is

Table 6.2 The coding schema and pathways of various GP computer systems across Britain.

Country	GP computer system	Context	Coding system	Total number of records	Unmatched codes	No code provided
Scotland	EMIS/Vision	Clinical events	Read v2	11.4 M	18k (0.2%)	0
		Prescription	Read v2	4.3 M	1 k	3.2 M (74%)
Wales	EMIS/Vision	Clinical events	Read v2	12.8 M	0	0
		Prescription	Read v2	7.5 M	0	0
England	Vision	Clinical events	Read v2	12 M	128k (1%)	0
		Prescription	Read v2	6.3 M	1 k	124k (2%)
	TPP	Clinical events	Read CTV3	87.5 M	2.5 M	0

approximately 70,000 items with a corresponding code. The BNF has an online and paper version that is updated annually via the NHS Business Services Authority. The BNF compromises chapters that have specific codes. Examples of this are shown in Table 6.3.

Table 6.3 The examples of how items are coded within the BNF.

BNF details	Character codes in the BNF	Exemplar code using Yaltormin SR 500 mg tablets	Description
Chapter	1 and 2	0601022BOBPAAAS	Chapter 6, endocrine system
Section	3 and 4	0601022BOBPAAAS	Drugs used in diabetes [38] (section 1)
Paragraph	5 and 6	0601022BOBPAAAS	Anti-diabetic drugs (paragraph 2)
Sub-paragraph	7	0601022BOBPAAAS	Biguanides (paragraph 2)
Product name	10 and 11	0601022BOBPAAAS	Yaltormin
Chemical substance	8 and 9	0601022BOBPAAAS	Metformin hydrochloride

Table 6.4 An example of a BNF code within Scottish primary care data.

Chapter length	Code	Estimated incidence	Details
Null	–	49k	–
1	3	Less than 10	Chapter
2	23	Less than 100	Codes associated with the chapter and those in the non0standard format are shown
4	0411	134k	Chapter and section

The method described above is demonstrated in specific way across all the different computer systems used in primary care. For example, in Scottish GP data, the standard BNF format is not always used. Most codes are shown with 15 characters and linked to the drug name and description. An example of a BNF code within Scottish primary care data is shown in Table 6.4.

The BNF codes within TPP extract show a basic format 00.00.00.00.00 where the coding structure cannot be mapped to codes provided by NHSBSA. The initial six digits of the code are usually related to the BNF chapter, section, and paragraph although inconsistencies have been detected. Therefore, to support any type of analysis or use within a clinical trial or epidemiology study, the BNF codes need to be described with specificity especially if multiple computer systems are used.

The prescription data within England are shown as a $dm+d$ code in patient medical records. The dm+d is a dictionary that was developed for use in primary and secondary care to code specific medicine and devices. These identifiers and text descriptions are useful to explore as part of big-data analysis and digital clinical trials. This method was highly important during the COVID-19 [39] pandemic to evaluate those who received vaccines versus those that did not, including any possible adverse events. The dm+d model has five specific components, as shown below:

- A virtual therapeutic moiety (VTM) is defined as the substance used in a patient's treatment
- An actual medicinal product (AMP) is defined as a single dose of a product linked to a specific manufacturer
- A virtual medicinal product (VMP) is defined as a group of properties in a single AMP
- A virtual medicinal product pack (VMPP) is defined as properties associated within one or more AMPPs
- An actual medicinal product pack (AMPP) is defined as a product supplied to be used directly by a patient

Table 6.5 An example of dm + d structure for Yaltormin 500 mg.

dm + d code	dm + d component	Description
109081006	VTM	Metformin
35547511000001101	AMP	Yaltormin SR 500 mg (Wockhardt UK Ltd)
386047000	VMP	Metformin 500 mg
8990611000001109	VMPP	Metformin 500 mg modified release tablets
35547811000001108	AMPP	Yaltormin SR 500 mg tables (Wockhardt UK Ltd)

Table 6.5 is an example of a dm+d structure for Yaltormin 500 mg. The product package comprises 56 tablets. In order to facilitate research studies, appropriate code lists have been generated from TRUD and NHSBSA. TRUD provided information on Read v2 and CTV3, in comparison to other coding systems although this is now being mapped to SNOMED CT. The accuracy of code lists therefore should be completed on a study-case basis by researchers who conduct the data extraction and analysis to ensure its authenticity. UK Biobank, for example, uses selected and validated codes to report health outcomes. This information is published in xx and the clinical code repository. Real-world data use is an important facet to optimise clinical practice; therefore, the notions of using clinically coded information in research are highly beneficial.

Hospital episode statistics (HES) is another set of data held by NHS Digital that can be linked to primary care data in England. Equivalent HES data in Scotland, Wales, and Northern Ireland can be used in a standardised format to answer various research questions including assessing quality outcome framework (QOF) and other factors. Primary and secondary care systems could have biases and fluctuations in errors due to human error, local processes, and procedures. Therefore, completeness and accuracy could be relative facets that need to be carefully addressed at the point of writing a statistical analysis plan which should specify extraction dates and cut-off points to address any missing data problems, mathematically.

Digital phenotyping

Digital phenotyping is a method that quantifies in situ of the clinical phenotypic data that may have been gathered from digital devices and EHRs. This method is still advancing as a clinical tool that could be routinely used in clinical practice. The use of aggregated data from smartphones and wearable technologies is another active port as activity and sensor measurement data could be used to generate categorical data that are not necessarily available within EHR systems. Data-driven objectivity is vital to support evidence-based medicine approaches that could act as a clinical utensil to treat more complex disease sequalae, for example. Whilst biological biomarkers remain the common choice, these can be rate limiting and digital biomarkers can be a solution to treating complex patients such as those with multi-morbidity. Widespread adoption of this has been demonstrated primarily within mental health [40] and pain medicine [41,42] research themes, as shown in Table 6.6.

Subtlety in symptoms and routine gathering of these is useful clinically as it can help with short, medium, and long-term clinical management. However, a common issue clinicians have is gaining access to these data in a timely manner and the reliability of self-

Table 6.6 Research themes and the digital phenotyping techniques used to address various themes.

Clinical theme	Disease	Digital phenotyping technique use	Examples
Mental health	Bipolar disorder	Used for ongoing symptom and relapse detection. Activity patterns including interaction with the digital application and metrics, including any voice measures could be used to determine depressive state. Relapse is a common issue among these patients; therefore, the data could also be used to predict these for patients with longitudinal data [43].	**Bipolar UK Mood Tracker** app which consists of a screening est. and a routine log to include medication use and dosage, etc. Notifications including reminders can be set.
	Addiction	Used for predicting relapse by way of a machine learning algorithm application using behaviour data obtained from smartphone sensors. An activity-based analysis over a time series is useful to also determine substance use relapse. A useful way to obtain this information could be via wearable devices that show triggers such as bars or liquor stores. This could also help develop relapse predictability and associated preventative interventions.	**Sure Recovery** app was designed to help with the addiction recovery journey; whether this be alcohol or other drugs. This has been used to track the recovery process from substance use and allows users to receive personalised text feedback and scores

Table 6.6 Research themes and the digital phenotyping techniques used to address various themes—cont'd

Clinical theme	Disease	Digital phenotyping technique use	Examples
	Suicidality	Multiple digital phenotypes could be gathered using smart phone based applications. Distinctive suicidal thoughts based on the intensity and variability is key to profile more severe and persistent thoughts could be used to prevent suicidality [44].	**Stay Alive** app was designed for those thinking about suicide or those worried about someone else feeling suicidal.
	Depression	Digital phenotyping improves the accuracy of depression diagnostics by way of measuring endophenotypes with ecological momentary assessments and the number of assessments completed over a period of time, including passive sensing that is gathered through the personal digital device [45].	**Headspace** app was designed for tracking depressive symptoms and supporting anyone with a depression diagnosis.
Pain medicine	Chronic pain	Opioid toxicity assessment by tracking dosage use. The use of a self-adherence tracker could prevent overdoses, respiratory failure associated with long-term use and addiction [46].	The **Second chance** app uses sonar to track breathing rates to detect an opioid overdose.
	Fibromialgia	Behavioural and pain event data are used to provide support. The digitally gathered data is used to provide support by way of information to improve pain management. The pain, medication and sleep tracker provide prediction of pain episodes and potential flare-ups.	**FMAUK Fibromapp** app
Obstetrics	Pre-eclampsia	Hypertension monitoring is key in pre-eclampsia. The app monitors the blood pressure and uses hypertension trends over a period of time to prompt suitable hospital visits [47].	**HaMpton** app
Neurology	Migraine	Tracking migraine attacks and the use of this to review patterns as well as triggers is the outcome of the phenotyping technique used within the app [46].	**Migraine Buddy** app
	Epilepsy	Self-monitoring technique used here includes the seizure safety checklist which is a clinical tool designed to assess risk and wellbeing.	**EpSMon or Epilepsy self monitor** app

Continued

Table 6.6 Research themes and the digital phenotyping techniques used to address various themes—cont'd

Clinical theme	Disease	Digital phenotyping technique use	Examples
Arthritis	Rheumatoid arthritis	Digital phenotyping method tracks the symptoms reported by patients which is summarised to prepare for clinical consultations. Appointments for a consultation could be prepared based on the summary reports.	RheumaBuddy app
Vascular medicine	Diabetes mellitus	The phenotypic characteristics of patients with diabetes are tracked including logging blood glucose levels and blood pressure. The data gathered could be summarised daily or weekly to adjust dietary intakes. Patients could share the recordings with healthcare professionals.	The Diabetes [38] UK Tracker app was designed for patients with Type 1 and Type 2 diabetes mellitus.
Respiratory medicine	Asthma	Senor technology is used to track exercise and peak flow ratings. The digital phenotype includes symptom-based alerts and triggers over a period of time. The sensor used in this app is CE marked [48].	Smart Peak Flow app is an asthma tracker and meter app

reporting as sometimes patients with complex clinical conditions may have difficulty with keeping up with self-monitoring. Other factors such as consistent use of medication for assessing adherence and the use of this data to reduce hospitalisations could also be useful facets to develop digital phenotyping methods.

6.5 Healthcare data regulations and governance

Healthcare data sharing and use require an array of governance oversight and approvals aligned to the current regulations. Raw data used for those patients that have not 'opted-out' can be used in clinical research. Thus, researchers and data providers alike should be clear about the data comprising those patients who are content to share their medical records for the purpose of research and education. This represents a fundamental requirement to respect patient consent and subsequent right to access their data.

The NHS needs to maintain trust with the general public and patients when providing the data using a secure platform. These are referred to as '*Trusted Research Environments*' (*TER*) or '*Secure Research Environment*' (*SRE*). The idea is that the TER and SREs are built and managed with minimal risks to data loss and protect against any data breaches. Building a TER can be challenging and sustainable management can be even more complex. The technical challenges that will need to be addressed on an ongoing basis include the competencies of the staff working within TREs require a deep knowledge base on data science, data architecture, clinical informatics, NHS data needs, and software development. It may be perceived that having a 'black-box' service may seem easier than procuring a TRE to conduct research. However, the 'black-box' approach also have disadvantages such as security issues with the changing governance and regulatory requirements in the United Kingdom, technical challenges such as embedding analytical tools required for specific study outputs, managing standardised working practices and codes.

TREs and SREs also have a clear governance arrangements and oversight with clear retention periods that are aligned to relevant research legislations. Therefore, data warehousing is another advantage to manage patient data in this way. As the data retained are also pseudonymised, this is likely to be in line with the common laws of the United Kingdom. The United Kingdom advises that the use of a TRE is a more suitable method to maintain a data platform. These usually have three specific components of a database service, a service wrapper, and a software specific to managing NHS data. Most service wrappers used have a permission framework for projects. These frameworks will have a clear privacy policy and governance framework built off the premise of a quality management system (QMS) that generates worklists and workflows for research staff involved with the study and the data processing team. The QMS prevents any inconsistencies and mishandling of the data used to deliver research projects.

6.6 Imaging data science [49–60]

There are several examples of innovations which have emerged from analytic and experimental design. Many studies published in high-impact journals have avoidable flaws in study design or methodology, which (potentially) could invalidate the results. Without doubt (and unfortunately), the most egregious examples are studies that employ imaging data sets that are too small to power a significant finding, for example, hundreds of parameters are evaluated but in only a couple dozen samples. There are other examples of analytical studies that are without validation and present models that are validated on the same data. Some studies have so-called 'information leakage' due to improper separation of training and validation data sets. A common example of this would be when the features are selected from the same data used to evaluate performance. Improper correction of multiple testing can bring a low p value or incorrect statistical outcome measures [1].

As these findings cannot be replicated, the credibility and perception of radiological data sets are threatened. There can be several reasons for this such as below:

I. Little or no formal background in imaging data set analysis and biostatistics
II. Lack of understanding of good study design
III. Lack of valid methods to arrive sound analytic results

Once these points are addressed, there is increased likelihood that another independent researcher will be able to replicate the results. Radiology and Nuclear Medicine data sets which are small in number can be correlated with pathological findings (which are considered gold standards) [61]. However, current software technologies are capable of extracting from imaging data, compounded by the complex relationships that exist between them, require the use of more sophisticated analytical methods (Fig. 6.3).

Radiomics and imaging data sets

Radiology, nuclear medicine, and multimodality hybrid medical images contain information which can reflect not only the current status but also the development and progression of disease process such as cancer. Extraction of several quantitative variables and conversion of medical images into minable data sets using comprehensive methods to analyse are known as Radiomics [2]. The extraction of data has evolved over time, initially high-dimensional quantitative features were used from CT, computed tomography (CT), magnetic resonance imaging (MRI), positron emission tomography (PET), and ultrasonography (US) [3], then the mining of correlations between these features and the diagnosis/prognosis of cancer [1,4]. A further analysis of these decoded data sets can reveal different imaging phenotypes [5].

There has been great progress within the field of Radiomics to increase the benefit of diagnostics and cancer treatment.

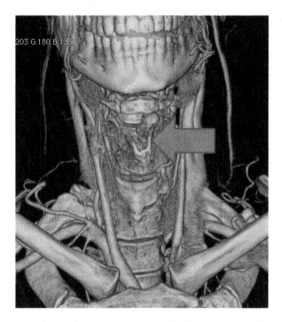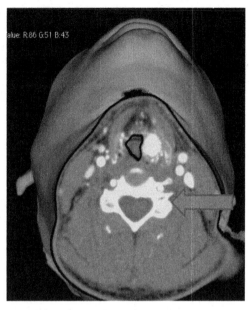

Fig. 6.3 3D reconstruction in patient with left-sided neck lump which was resected and diagnosed as paraganglioma. 3D images are often read in conjunction with axial images. The images can be superimposed on each other, i.e. 2D image overlaid on a 3D image for better understanding of anatomical location of pathology.

Radiomics has brought in a new way to extract data in the medical images which in the past were only considered as static images for visual inspection only and relied on the skill of the reader. This has resulted in advancement in precision diagnostics, outlook of cancer, and cancer treatment [6]. Radiomics achieves this by obtaining quantitative information from medical images, combining imaging features with clinical information, genomic information, and other information, and mining these data to detect radiomic biomarkers [7].

Importance of imaging informatics and imaging data set science in radiology and nuclear medicine

Artificial intelligence, data science, and clinical informatics have been covered in detail in Chapter 6 of the book. Here, we are briefly discussing the importance of imaging informatics and imaging data sets related to diagnostic Radiology and Nuclear Medicine.

An 'imaging informaticist' is a unique individual who sits at the intersection of clinical radiology, data science, and information technology. As the informaticist has the ability to understand each of the different domains and translate between the experts in these domains, imaging informaticists are now essential players in the development, evaluation, and deployment of AI in the clinical environment [8]. There three important domains covered by imaging informaticists:

(1) Data curation
(2) Processing
(3) Labelling
(4) Deidentification

The labels need to be reviewed for consistency and quality before an algorithm is used. These problems are tackled in imaging informatics. Following are some useful terminologies for the beginner to benchmark the quality assurance steps.

(a) Digital Imaging Adoption Model (DIAM): a collaboration between three major imaging informatics societies
(b) The Annotation and Image Mark up (AIM) Project: Introduction of standardised format for annotations created on medical images
(c) Protected Health Information (PHI): Information embedded within the imaging data such as DICOM tags, the facial reconstruction ability, identification of jewellery, etc.
(d) Society of Imaging Informatics Workflow Initiative (SWIM): Identification of workflow steps and addressing inaccuracies of manually created timestamps.

Radiologists, nuclear medicine physicians, and imaging informaticists contribute to the development of imaging-based artificial intelligence tools. These not only evaluate the results but also check for accuracy and likelihood of successful deployment in the clinical workflow. One of the best example of quality work which has clinical impact throughout the world is related to Nuclear Medicine Cardiac work done at the Cidar Sinai Medical Imaging Centre [9] (Fig. 6.4).

Non-invasive quantification of ischaemia is now a reality and used in clinical domain very commonly. Variables such as ejection fraction, percentage of ischaemia, left ventricular volume, left ventricular diastolic and systolic data sets, and shape of the heart can be derived with one click of a button.

Imaging data sets and international imaging societies

American College of Radiology, Radiological Society of North America, Royal College of Radiologists, and several other societies

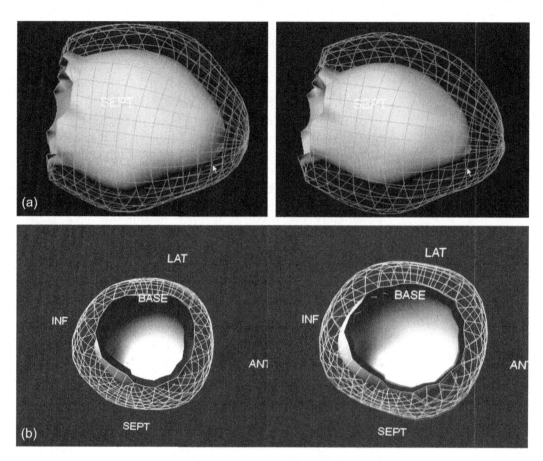

Fig. 6.4 3D surface contouring of heart using software models following myocardial perfusion scan for evaluation of ischaemic heart disease. *Top row* contains images in diastolic and systolic phase while *bottom row* contains image demonstrating the contours of the heart from the base.

are working to establish a range of initiatives to address the need for quality imaging data sets [10].

I. The RadLex Vocabulary (RadLex.org)
II. Radiology Report Templates (RadReport.org)
III. Radelements (radelement.org)

As a result of efforts of cooperative clinical subspecialty societies, industry, and regulatory bodies, there is active development of the infrastructure, formats, and data structures. The main purpose is to obtain the most information possible from the massive amount of digital medical image data now available. This new infrastructure aims to empower universal access to the next wave of radiologists' tools. These tools will be based on standardised, quantitative measurements and descriptions and computer algorithms capable of finding patterns in data that are beyond current abilities.

Imaging data sets and language of 3D imaging

Multi-detector row CT scans have the capability to create images in planes other than axial images traditionally used for image interpretation. Although the 3D data sets improve the utility of DICOM data set for understanding but can also create confusion when trying to describe a method or an image. Post processing cannot be optimised unless innovating imaging parameters are used to display voluminous data [11]. For researchers, there are some basic terminologies which should be understood before manipulating CT data to create multiplanar and 3D images.

Collimation

The act of controlling the beam size with a metallic aperture near the tube. This determines the amount of tissue exposed as the X-ray beam rotates around the patient.

Beam collimation

The application of same concept of collimation from single-detector row CT to multi-detector row CT. Multiple channels of data are acquired simultaneously.

I. Narrow collimation: Only the central small detector elements are exposed.
II. Wider collimation: This may expose the entire detector array.

Section collimation

Partition of incident X-ray beam into multiple subdivided channels of data. Compared with beam collimation which determines volume coverage, section collimation determines minimal section thickness that can be reconstructed.

Data reconstruction

The process of generating axial images from projection data is referred to as data reconstruction in the context of Radiology. This is a mathematical process that utilises different angles leading to the final image quality and radiation dose. Iterative reconstruction

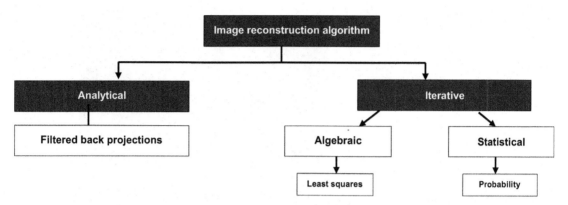

Fig. 6.5 How pathways for data reconstructing, including iterative reconstruction.

can be completed using different imaging techniques although a common method would be to use an iterative algorithm, which can be applied to both 2D and 3D images (Fig. 6.5).

Section thickness and interval

This is the length of each segment of data along the z axis during data reconstruction. This defines the volume of tissue that will be included in the calculation to generate the Hounsfield unit value assigned to each of the pixels that make up the image. Interval refers to the distance between the centre of one transverse reconstruction and the next.

Volumetric data set

A thin-section data set can be generated in addition to or in place of axial images. These are called volumetric data sets. These are not intended for axial image interpretation but for generating multiplanar reformatted or volume rendered images, usually 1 mm or less section thickness and preferably overlapping interval.

Multiplanar reconstruction (MPR)

This is the process of using data from axial CT images to create non-axial 2D image in coronal, sagittal, oblique, or curved plane generated from only one voxel in thickness transecting a set or stack of axial images (Fig. 6.6).

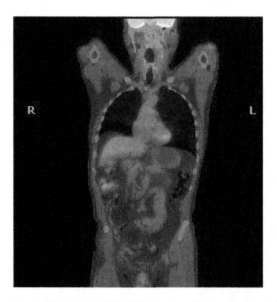

Fig. 6.6 Coral-fused PET CT with 18F FDG (fluorine-18 fluorodeoxyglucose) as a biomarker. This biomarker is used most commonly for molecular imaging of cancer. The scan consists of a low-dose CT scan and a positron emission tomography (PET) scan superimposed on each other for better anatomical and functional delineation of abnormalities.

Maximum intensity projection images (MIP)

MIP images display only the highest attenuation value from data. These are most useful when objects of interest are the brightest objects in the image (Fig. 6.7).

Shaded surface display

These are also called surface rendered images and provide a 3D view of the surface of an object (Fig. 6.8).

Volume-rendered image

3D images are reconstructed using opacity value and lighting effects to allow appreciation of spatial relationships between structures. These images use the rapid data processing inherent in the human optical pathways to achieve intuitive perception of depth relationships in large data sets.

It is necessary to understand the strength and weaknesses of available imaging processing techniques. A good example is CT colonography which is a non-invasive way or assessing bowel

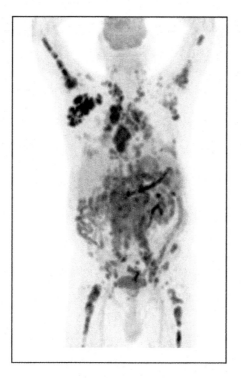

Fig. 6.7 Maximum Intensity Projection (MIP) image: There is widespread metabolically active nodal disease above and below the level of diaphragm. The most metabolically active nodes are seen in the chest and right axilla. There is also metabolically active disease in the bone marrow in keeping with infiltration. The MIP image facilitates understanding of aggressive nature of cancer and also to target a site for biopsy which in this case would be right axilla under ultrasound guidance.

lumen and the 3D capability can be used to integrate real-time rendering into routine image interpretation.

Clinical Radiology and Nuclear Medicine as molecular imaging specialities are faced with potentially the most disruptive technology it has ever encountered. This challenge refers to 'data science', 'artificial intelligence', 'big data, etc. which has the potential to change the essence of what it means to be a Radiologist, Nuclear medicine physician, or a Radionuclide Radiologist (12). This change is not just a cosmetic change to the imaging specialities. Most of the imaging journals have now added articles related to 'Data Science'. Radiological Society of North America has started a new journal related to Artificial Intelligence. JACR has added Data Science to the cover as a new pillar. Special issues on 'Data Science' are being published. These special issues act as primer

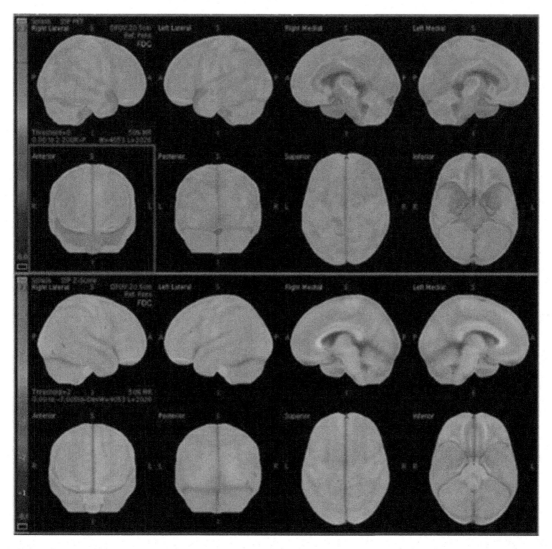

Fig. 6.8 Alzheimer's disease. 3D Axial grey-scale FDG PET images *(bottom row)* and 3D stereotactic surface projection (SSP) images *(top row)* demonstrate bilateral hypometabolism in the parietotemporal cortices *(red colour; dark grey in print versions)* and in the posterior cingulate–precuneus cortices (a pattern that is typical of Alzheimer's disease). The 3D image display shows one of the earliest signs of Alzheimer's disease which is related to reduced metabolism in the posterior cingulate gyrus hypometabolism.

for the new starters. The British Institute of Radiology is organising 'Artificial Intelligence Study days' (Fig. 6.9).

There are now open calls for manuscripts to authors known to be working in this subject area. The editorial teams of journals have included appointment of editors with special interest in data

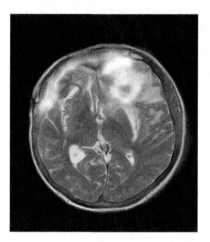

Fig. 6.9 18F Choline Brain PET-MR image in a patient with post treatment glioma. The avid area in the left frontal lobe shows residual area of tumour. With selection of right data sets and use of hybrid imaging techniques several physiological processes can be mapped. In this case using 18F Choline as a biomarker, the process of cell membrane multiplication has been imaged.

science [12]. All these may seem an overkill at present, but there is far-reaching role 'data science' will play in the future of imaging modalities. This is only start of an exercise which will make readers better equipped to deal with the challenges and opportunities by this rapidly advancing field.

6.7 Big data

In the current context, *Big data* can be defined as significant amounts of structured data (tables, spreadsheets, databases with columns and rows, CSV, and Excel), or unstructured (email, social media, text, customer habits, smartphones, GPS, websites, etc.). Typically, these data have been stored in the cloud or in data centres, which are then used by companies, organisations, universities, startups, and even the government, for different purposes [62].

Big data is commonly associated with other areas such as machine learning, data science, AI, and deep learning. As these fields of analysis still require the reading and analysis of data, big data will continue to play an important role in improving existing models and will allow advances in research. In the context of clinical imaging, Big data comprises large quantities of images of organs and tissue gathered in '*slice*' formation.

Case study

Paragangliomas are cells of neural origin. These belong to the group of neuroendocrine tumours (although more common in women with a ratio of 3:1) [1,2]. Majority of cases present with symptoms of hoarseness, haemoptysis, and airway compromise. Functioning glottic paragangliomas are very rare [3]. Although majority of the laryngeal Paragangliomas are rare, historical literature has suggested 25% of malignant tumours (inclusive of neuroendocrine carcinomas) [4].

The paragangliomas are divided broadly into two main groups [5]:

(a) Epithelial origin: well-differentiated (rare), moderately differentiated, and poorly differentiated subtypes (more common).

(b) Neural origin

We describe a case of supraglottic paraganglioma highlighting the importance of multimodality imaging. With advancements in anatomical and functional imaging, it is anticipated that the use of 'simultaneous MR/PET' imaging will prove to be extremely useful for characterising these lesions.

A 43-year-old man presented with 2 months' history of dragging sensation in his throat and slight difficulty in deep breathing. He had 3 years' history of hoarseness of his voice. The hoarseness was intermittent initially but gradually became constant. He denied shortness of breath at rest but occasionally used to wake up at night short of breath. He denied any weight loss. There was no significant past medical history. He was on Sertaraline and Clonazepam for a chronic fatigue disorder. He smoked 3–5 times per day for 6 years. He had an occasional alcohol intake.

On endoscopic examination, there was a very large mass on the left side of his vocal fold in the larynx. Neck ultrasound showed a well-defined mass in the left supraglottic region with no obvious cartilage invasion. No cervical lymphadenopathy was noted. Flexible nasendoscopy (Fig. 6.10) revealed a swelling in the left supraglottic region which appeared very smooth and spherical with partial obstruction of the airway.

MRI confirmed this to be a 19-mm supraglottic mass (Fig. 6.13).

I-123 MIBG scans (Fig. 6.14) were obtained at 4 h and 24 h post injection which showed no focal uptake in the neck.

18F FDG PET/CT showed a solitary focus of increased FDG uptake (SUV max 9.3) (Fig. 6.15A) in the left supraglottic region, measuring approximately 19 mm × 11 mm. This mass was also Gallium Octreotate avid on subsequent PET/CT (SUV max 116) (Fig. 6.15B). Physiological distribution of FDG and Gallium Octreotate was seen elsewhere. The Gallium Octreotate PET and MR images were fused manually using Advantage workstation (ADW 4.4 and Osirix) (Fig. 6.16).

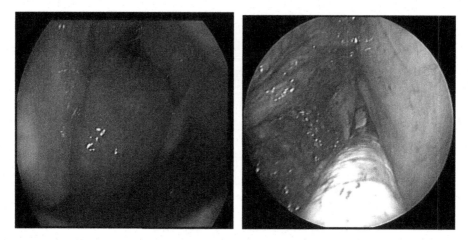

Fig. 6.10 Endoscopic view of the supraglottic region which shows a smooth well-defined soft tissue mass (as viewed from above) along the wall of the laryngo-pharynx. Contrast-enhanced CT of the neck shows enhancing mass with blood supply from a branch of left internal carotid artery (Figs 6.11 and 6.12).

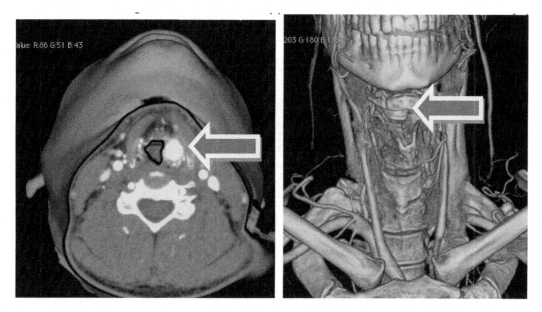

Fig. 6.11 Axial contrast-enhanced CT fused with 3D surface rendering overlay image showing an enhancing mass at the lateral wall of the glottic region. *Arrow head* on 3D skeleton view shows the supraglottic location of the mass.

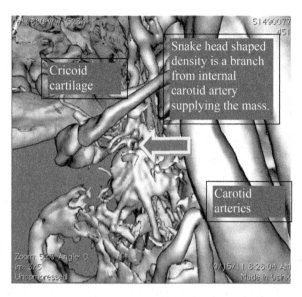

Fig. 6.12 Zoomed view of the lateral part of the CT Neck Angiogram. The pillars on the left are the carotid vessels and jugular vein. There is a serpinginous (snake head)-shaped density entering the superior aspect of the mass *(arrow head)*. The mass is supplied by a branch of internal carotid artery.

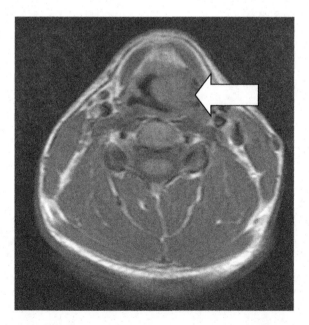

Fig. 6.13 Axial T1W MRI scan through the neck showing a soft tissue mass which is low to intermediate signal occupying left lateral wall of the laryngo-pharynx.

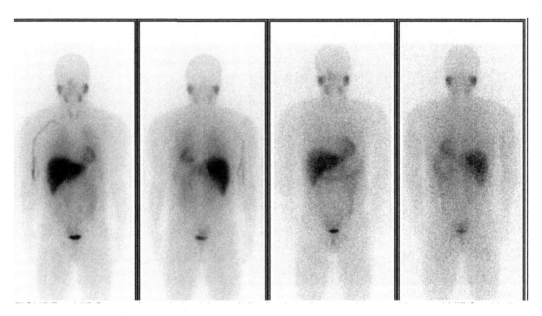

Fig. 6.14 MIBG scan shows physiological distribution of tracer with no evidence of MIBG avid disease in the neck.

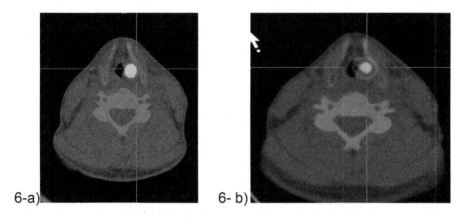

6-a) 6- b)

Fig. 6.15 (A) Axial fused Gallium 68 Octreotate PET/CT and (B) axial fused 18F FDG PET/CT demonstrating tracer avid soft tissue mass on the medial aspect of the left thyroid cartilage which is more avid on Gallium Octreotate PET/CT.

The anatomical and functional imaging raised the possibility of a neuro-endocrine tumour. The mass was excised with CO_2 laser at 10 watts. Intra-operatively there was a bleeding episode, and decision

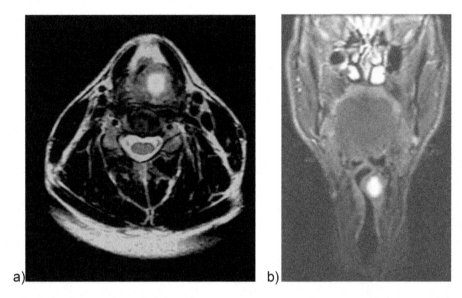

a)   b)

Fig. 6.16 Sequential MR/PET of the neck (A) Axial T2 MRI and Gallium 68 Octreotate PET fusion and (B) Coronal fat-suppressed MRI and Gallium 68 Octreotate PET fusion showing tracer avid soft tissue abnormality in the supraglottic region.

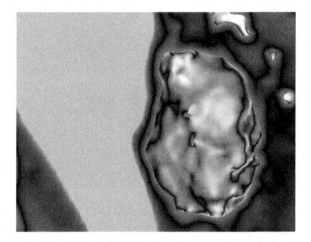

Fig. 6.17 Zoomed 3D surface rendering Gallium Octreotate PET/CT of the laryngo-pharynx showing soft tissue mass which is compressing the wall of the larynx. The 'glow' from the mass represents Somatostatin receptor positive status – a feature of neuroendocrine tumours.

was made to ligate the supraglottic blood vessels. He made smooth recovery post-operatively. The histopathology confirmed this soft tissue mass to be laryngeal paraganglioma (Fig. 6.17).

Learning objectives

Histologically, controversy exists about the diagnostic features of paraganglioma as classic histopathological finding of 'Zellballen pattern' (chief cells clustered into round group of nest cells) can also be seen in carcinoid tumours, melanomas, and medullary carcinoma of the thyroid [6]. This problem is further complicated by the anatomical fact that moderately differentiated paragangliomas prove to be a diagnostic and therapeutic challenge due to extreme vascularity and pre-operative optimum diagnostic approaches have been suggested to avoid complications related to bleeding [7].

Preoperative evaluation of these lesions should include use of a contrast agent to assess the vascularity of these lesions (as seen in this case). MRI has advantage of outlining the anatomical boundaries of soft tissue tumours better than other imaging modalities. Use of MRI helps to assess the exact anatomical location and possible invasion of deeper structures.

With advancements in anatomical and molecular imaging techniques, Gallium 68 DOTATATE PET/CT has proven to be a novel imaging modality, and it has been reported to be superior to 18F FDG PET CT for imaging well-differentiated neuroendocrine tumours [8]. The technique utilises a distinct property of neuroendocrine tumours as they express high-density somatostatin receptors at the cell membrane. This facilitates the use of radiolabeled somatostatin analogues for imaging of these tumours [9]. Although these tumours may be low-grade and less avid on 18F FDG PET, combined use of 18F FDG PET/CT and Ga 68 PET/CT improves the overall diagnostic performance when compared with either tracer [8].

At molecular levels, these tumours can be investigate by use of I-123 MIBG (meta-iodo-benzyl-guanidine), 18F FDG PET/CT, and Gallium 68 PET/CT. Depending upon underlying receptor status, these lesions may be avid on all or one of the imaging modalities.

The use of combined anatomical and molecular imaging has seen remarkable developments in the recent past. Scientists and physicists have been working hard to develop a common tool where best possible anatomical imaging could be combined with the best possible molecular imaging techniques. The result of this combined effort is evolution of PET/MRI scanning.

PET/MRI scanning can be done in two forms:

(a) Sequential PET/MRI: scans obtained on two different scanners and fused utilising software on workstations

(b) Simultaneous PET/MRI: scans obtained on a single machine at the same time.

We have utilised the sequential MR/PET imaging and have highlighted that the sequential MR/PET has the ability to characterise salient features of these tumours on a single test, i.e. anatomical configuration, invasion of surrounding tissues, vascularity with use of contrast agent, and last but not the least, the receptor status. It is anticipated that the use of 'Simultaneous PET/MRI' imaging will facilitate lesion analysis and optimise therapeutic approach for safer management of these patients.

Paragangliomas are tumours of neural origin which can have varied clinical presentation and [63] histopathological features. It is prudent to optimise pre-operative evaluation of these tumours so as to avoid complications and channelize the therapeutic options. Combined anatomical and functional imaging modalities such as PET/MRI would optimise patient care and facilitate diagnosis of these lesions.

References

[1] Provost F, Fawcett T. Data science and its relationship to big data and data-driven decision making. Big Data 2013;1(1):51–9. https://doi.org/10.1089/big.2013.1508.

[2] Sanchez-Pinto LN, Luo Y, Churpek MM. Big data and data science in critical care. Chest 2018;154(5):1239–48. https://doi.org/10.1016/j.chest.2018.04.037.

[3] Lähnemann D, Köster J, Szczurek E, McCarthy DJ, Hicks SC, Robinson MD, et al. Eleven grand challenges in single-cell data science. Genome Biol 2020;21(1):31. https://doi.org/10.1186/s13059-020-1926-6.

[4] Zhang X, Pérez-Stable EJ, Bourne PE, Peprah E, Duru OK, Breen N, et al. Big data science: opportunities and challenges to address minority health and health disparities in the 21st century. Ethnicity Disease 2017;27(2):95–106. https://doi.org/10.18865/ed.27.2.95.

[5] Larry Fennigkoh D. Courtney Nanney; CMMSs de mineração de dados: como converter dados em conhecimento. Biomed Instrument Technol 2018;52 (s2):28–33. https://doi.org/10.2345/0899-8205-52.s2.28.

[6] Ayanian JZ, Landon BE, Newhouse JP, Zaslavsky AM. Racial and ethnic disparities among enrollees in medicare advantage plans. N Engl J Med 2014;371 (24):2288–97. https://doi.org/10.1056/NEJMsa1407273.

[7] Office of the National Coordinator for Health Information Technology. Percent of REC enrolled providers in an organization/site and area type live on an EHR and demonstrating meaningful use. Washington, DC: Office of the National Coordinator for Health Information; 2016.

[8] Obama B. United States health care reform: progress to date and next steps. JAMA 2016;316(5):525–32. https://doi.org/10.1001/jama.2016.9797.

[9] Chapter 11: Knowledge and Information Ethics Department of Computer Science, City University of New York, New York, USA. Department of Health, University of Medicine and Dentistry, New Jersey, USA n.d.

[10] Yin H, Fan F, Zhang J, Li H, Lau TF. The Importance of Domain Knowledge. Retrieved from: http://blog.ml.cmu.edu/2020/08/31/1-domain-knowledge/#:~:text=Precise%20and%20accurate%20problem%20definition,how%20users%20browse%20online-stores.

[11] Waller MA, Fawcett SE. Data science, predictive analytics, and big data: a revolution that will transform supply chain design and management. J Bus Logist 2013;34:77–84. https://doi.org/10.1111/jbl.12010.

[12] National Academies of Sciences, Engineering, and Medicine; Division of Behavioral and Social Sciences and Education; Board on Science Education; Division on Engineering and Physical Sciences; Committee on Applied and Theoretical Statistics; Board on Mathematical Sciences and Analytics, et al. Data Science for Undergraduates: Opportunities and Options. Washington (DC): National Academies Press (US); 2018. p. 2. Knowledge for Data Scientists. Available from: https://www.ncbi.nlm.nih.gov/books/NBK532764.

[13] Forbes CL. IBM predicts demand for data scientists will soar 28% by 2020; 2017.

[14] CRA (Computing Research Association). Computing Research and the Emerging Field of Data Science; 2016.

[15] Codella NCF, Nguyen QB, Pankanti S, Gutman D, Helba B, Halpern A, et al. Deep learning ensembles for melanoma recognition in dermoscopy images. IBM J Res Dev 2017;61(4):1–15. https://doi.org/10.48550/arXiv.1610.04662.

[16] Chen H, Chiang RHL, Storey VC. Business intelligence and analytics: from big data to big impact. MIS Q 2012;36(4):1165–88. https://doi.org/10.2307/41703503.

[17] Kitchin R. The real-time city? Big data and smart urbanism. GeoJournal 2014;79:1–14. https://doi.org/10.1007/s10708-013-9516-8.

[18] Bouamrane M-M, Rector A, Hurrell M. Experience of using OWL ontologies for automated inference of routine pre-operative screening tests the semantic web - ISWC 2010. Berlin: Springer Berlin Heidelberg; 2010.

[19] Tao C, Solbrig H, Sharma D, Wei W-Q, Savova G, Chute C. Time-oriented question answering from clinical narratives using semantic-web techniques. The semantic web - ISWC 2010. Berlin: Springer Berlin Heidelberg; 2010.

[20] Bouamrane M-M, Tao C. Managing interoperability and compleXity in health systems. In: MIXHS'11 Proceedings of the 20th ACM international conference on information and knowledge management, CIKM'11, Glasgow; 2011. p. 2635–6.

[21] Tao C, Bouamrane M-M. Managing interoperability and compleXity in health systems. In: MIXHS'12 proceedings of the 21st ACM international conference on information and knowledge management, CIKM'12, Maui, Hawaii; 2012. p. 2758–9.

[22] Gibbons P, Arzt N, Burke-Beebe S, Chute C, Dickinson G, Flewelling T, et al. Coming to terms: scoping interoperability in health care. Health level seven EHR interoperability work group, 2007. Retrieved from: https://www.hln.com/assets/pdf/Coming-to-Terms-February-2007.pdf.

[23] Benson T. Principles of health interoperability HL7 and SNOMED. Health informatics series. Berlin: Springer; 2010.

[24] McGee-Lennon M, Bouamrane M-M, Barry S, et al. Evaluating the delivery of assisted living lifestyles at scale (Dallas). In: Proceedings of HCI 2012 - People & Computers XXVI, The 26th BCS Conference on Human Computer Interaction, Birmingham; 12–14 September; 2012.

[25] Fridsma D. Interoperability vs health information exchange: setting the record straight 2013. Available from: https://www.healthit.gov/buzz-blog/meaningful-use/interoperability-healthinformation-exchange-setting-record-straight/.

[26] Benson T. Principles of health interoperability HL7 and SNOMED2010. London: Springer; 2010.

[27] Health Information and Quality Authority Overview of Healthcare Interoperability Standards., 2013. Available from: https://www.hiqa.ie/system/files/Healthcare-Interoperability-Standards.pdf.

[28] Delanerolle G, Zeng Y, Phiri P, Phan T, Tempest N, Busuulwa P, et al. Systematic review and meta-analysis of mental health impact on BAME populations with preterm birth. medRxiv 2022. https://doi.org/10.1101/2022.03.22.22272780.

[29] Berners-Lee T, Hendler J, Lassila O. The semantic web. Sci Am 2001;284:34–43.

[30] Cambridge Semantics. Semantic University. Available from: https://cambridgesemantics.com/blog/semantic-university/comparing-semantic-technologies/.

[31] Tsang RSM, Joy M, Whitaker H, Sheppard JP, Williams J, Sherlock J, et al. Development and validation of a modified Cambridge Multimorbidity Score for use with internationally recognized electronic health record clinical terms (SNOMED CT). medRxiv 2022;, 22271765. https://doi.org/10.1101/2022.03.02.22271765.

[32] Delanerolle G, Williams R, Stipancic A, Byford R, Forbes A, Anand S, et al. Methodological issues for using a common data model (CDM) of COVID-19 vaccine uptake and important adverse events of interest (AEIs): the Data and Connectivity COVID-19 Vaccines Pharmacovigilance (DaC-VaP) United Kingdom feasibility study. JMIR Preprints 2022;, 37821.

[33] Centers for Disease Control and Prevent. ICD-10-CM Codes File, www.cdc.gov/nchs/data/icd/icd10cm_fy_2017_codes_file.pdf. [Accessed 22 June 2022].

[34] Hohl CM, Karpov A, Reddekopp L, Doyle-Waters M, Stausberg J. ICD-10 codes used to identify adverse drug events in administrative data: a systematic review. J Am Med Inform Assoc 2014;21(3):547–57. https://doi.org/10.1136/amiajnl-2013-002116. Erratum in: J Am Med Inform Assoc 2014;21(4):757. Doyle-Waters, Mimi [added].

[35] DuvaSawko. Consequences of Medical Coding & Billing Errors & How to Avoid Them, www.duvasawko.com/medical-coding-errors/. [Accessed 22 June 2022].

[36] ICD-10-CM Abbreviations. NEC, NOSby Christine Woolstenhulme, QCC, QMCS, CPC, CMRS., 2015, https://www.findacode.com/articles/icd-10-cm-abbreviations-nec-nos-31650.html. [Accessed 22 June 2022].

[37] 2022 ICD-10-CM Diagnosis Code E08.9, https://www.icd10data.com/ICD10CM/Codes/E00-E89/E08-E13/E08-/E08.9. [Accessed 22 June 2022].

[38] Heald AH, Jenkins DA, Chaudhury N, Williams R, Sperrin M, Peek N, et al. Application of a city wide digital population database for outcome analysis in diabetes: SARS-CoV-2, diabetes and hospital admission rate month by month in Greater Manchester, UK. Cardiovasc Endocrinol Metab 2022;11(1), e0257. https://doi.org/10.1097/xce.0000000000000257.

[39] Heald AH, Jenkins DA, Chaudhury N, Williams R, Sperrin M, Peek N, et al. SARS-CoV-2, diabetes and mortality: month by month variation in mortality rate from June 2020 to June 2021. Cardiovasc Endocrinol Metab 2022;11(1), e0258. https://doi.org/10.1097/xce.0000000000000258.

[40] Delanerolle G, Ayis S, Barzilova V, Phiri P, Zeng Y, Ranaweera S, et al. A systematic review and meta-analysis of polycystic ovary syndrome and mental health among Black Asian minority ethnic populations. medRxiv 2022;, 22271948. https://doi.org/10.1101/2022.03.05.22271948.

[41] Shetty A, Delanerolle G, Zeng Y, Shi JQ, Ebrahim R, Pang J, et al. A systematic review and meta-analysis of digital application use in clinical research in pain medicine. MedRxiv 2022;, 22271773. https://doi.org/10.1101/2022.03.02.22271773.

[42] Latif M, Awan F, Gul M, Husain M, Husain M, Sayyed K, et al. Preliminary evaluation of a culturally adapted CBT-based online programme for depression and anxiety from a lower middle-income country. Cogn Behav Ther 2021;14, E36. https://doi.org/10.1017/S1754470X21000313.

[43] Hsu M, Ahern DK, Suzuki J. Digital phenotyping to enhance substance use treatment during the COVID-19 pandemic. JMIR Ment Health 2020;7(10): e21814.

[44] Kleiman EM, Turner BJ, Fedor S, Beale EE, Picard RW, Huffman JC, Nock MK. Digital phenotyping of suicidal thoughts. Depress Anxiety 2018;35(7):601–8. https://doi.org/10.1002/da.22730.

[45] Kamath J, et al. Digital phenotyping in depression diagnostics: integrating psychiatric and engineering perspectives. World J Psychiatry 2022;12:393–409. https://doi.org/10.5498/wjp.v12.i3.393.

[46] The #1 Migraine & Headache Tracking App, https://migrainebuddy.com/. [Accessed 22 June 2022].

[47] http://www.asmakhalil.co.uk/hampton-about-the-app/.

[48] Smart Peak Flow: Asthma Diary, https://www.blf.org.uk/technology-for-lung-health/smart-peak-flow-asthma-diary. [Accessed 22 June 2022].

[49] Aerts HJWL. Data science in radiology: a path forward. Clin Cancer Res 2018;24(3):532–4. https://doi.org/10.1158/1078-0432.ccr-17-2804.

[50] Liu Z, Wang S, Dong D, Wei J, Fang C, Zhou X, et al. The applications of radiomics in precision diagnosis and treatment of oncology: opportunities and challenges. Theranostics 2019;9(5):1303–22. https://doi.org/10.7150/thno.30309.

[51] Kumar V, Gu Y, Basu S, Berglund A, Eschrich SA, Schabath MB, et al. Radiomics: the process and the challenges. Magn Reson Imaging 2012;30 (9):1234–48. https://doi.org/10.1016/j.mri.2012.06.010.

[52] Gatenby RA, Grove O, Gillies RJ. Quantitative imaging in cancer evolution and ecology. Radiology 2013;269(1):8–15. https://doi.org/10.1148/radiol.13122697.

[53] Aerts HJWL. The potential of radiomic-based phenotyping in precision medicine: a review. JAMA Oncol 2016;2(12):1636–42. https://doi.org/10.1001/jamaoncol.2016.2631.

[54] Lambin P, Leijenaar RTH, Deist TM, Peerlings J, de Jong EEC, van Timmeren J, et al. Radiomics: the bridge between medical imaging and personalized medicine. Nat Rev Clin Oncol 2017;14(12):749–62. https://doi.org/10.1038/nrclinonc.2017.141.

[55] El Naqa I, Grigsby P, Apte A, Kidd E, Donnelly E, Khullar D, et al. Exploring feature-based approaches in PET images for predicting cancer treatment outcomes. Pattern Recognit 2009;42(6):1162–71. https://doi.org/10.1016/j.patcog.2008.08.011.

[56] Cook TS. The importance of imaging informatics and informaticists in the implementation of AI. Acad Radiol 2020;27(1):113–6. https://doi.org/10.1016/j.acra.2019.10.002.

[57] Slomka PJ, Miller RJH, Hu L-H, Germano G, Berman DS. Solid-state detector SPECT myocardial perfusion imaging. J Nucl Med 2019;60(9):1194–204. https://doi.org/10.2967/jnumed.118.220657.

[58] Kohli M, Alkasab T, Wang K, Heilbrun ME, Flanders AE, Dreyer K, et al. Bending the artificial intelligence curve for radiology: informatics tools from ACR and RSNA. J Am Coll Radiol 2019;16(10):1464–70. https://doi.org/10.1016/j.jacr.2019.06.009.

[59] Dalrymple NC, Prasad SR, Freckleton MW, Chintapalli KN. Informatics in radiology (infoRAD): introduction to the language of three-dimensional

imaging with multidetector CT. Radiographics 2005;25(5):1409–28. https://doi.org/10.1148/rg.255055044.

[60] Hillman BJ. Data science and the future of radiology: a new pillar for JACR. J Am Coll Radiol 2018;15(3):378. https://doi.org/10.1016/j.jacr.2017.12.005.

[61] Delanerolle G, Cavalini H, Phiri P, Gelling L. A scoping systematic review of implementation frameworks to effectively transition interventions into clinical practice in oncology, nuclear medicine and radiology. MedRxiv 2022;, 22271946. https://doi.org/10.1101/2022.03.05.22271946.

[62] John Hopkins DS Specialization Series. Big Data: Its Benefits, Challenges, and Future. A brief look at Big Data and the future., 2020, https://towardsdatascience.com/big-data-its-benefits-challenges-and-future-6fddd69ab927. [Accessed 8 March 2022].

[63] Meza-Torres B, Delanerolle G, Okusi C, Mayer N, Anand S, McCartney J, et al. Differences in clinical presentation with long covid following community and hospital infection, and associations with all-cause mortality: English sentinel network database study. JMIR Preprints 2022;, 37668.

Further reading

Tsang RSM, Joy M, Whitaker H, Sheppard JP, Williams J, Sherlock J, Mayor N, Meza-Torres B, Button E, Williams AJ, Kar D, Delanerolle G, McManus R, Hobbs FDR, de Lusignan S. Development and validation of a modified Cambridge Multimorbidity Score for use with internationally recognized electronic health record clinical terms (SNOMED CT). medRxiv 2022;, 22271765. https://doi.org/10.1101/2022.03.02.22271765.

7

Organisational structure and research readiness

Key messages

- Organisation structure with transparent reporting and management models are important.
- Research readiness involves a five-step procedure in the United Kingdom including, but not limited to taking stock, a well-designed research strategy, regular re-evaluation of existing infrastructure, and research resourcing architecture, emphasising the use of novel digital technologies and relevant standard and, regular training for all research staff.
- Matrix management styles should be considered to develop organisation structure and research readiness.
- Develop and maintain guidelines for readiness levels specific to clinical specialties to ensure that consistent approaches are used to across the United Kingdom.

7.1   Introduction

Conceptualisation of organisation structure and associated hierarchy is a manifestation of systematic processes comprising of thoughts, relationships between elements, and the systems in place. Whilst definitions of structures vary, depending on the type of organisation discussed, a general overview would refer to the relationship between the components of an organised entity embedded within a framework comprising a variety of elements. In the context of research, operational structure and deliverability of studies are influenced by the type of organisation and structure available in a specific geographical location. As a result of this, healthcare organisations, commercial entities, charitable organisations, independent research institutions, and academic organisations conduct research differently.

Clinical Trials and Tribulations. https://doi.org/10.1016/B978-0-12-821787-0.00001-5

Organisational structure

Organisational theory is the premise to organisational structure as it sets the propositions for organisation science where the study of institutional practice occurs. These practices are examined through research to develop knowledge that could aid in understanding practices and improve elements of the institutional environment. Organisational structure definitions have evolved over the years. More established definitions describe an organisational structure using a framework. Mintzberg [1] reported an organisational structure to comprise a framework that demonstrated the relationship between systems, processes, people, jobs, and groups that function for a common goal. Organisational structure lacks a coordination mechanism which impacts organisation processes, thus models of internal relationism, power, reporting hierarchy, formalities such as communication methods, responsibility, and decision-making are part of an organisation structure's definition. Arnold and Feldman [2] reported that organisational structure is defined as a formal information flow model that uses a facility. These definitions have similarities, and the representation of the concepts is based on two principles of process and relationship between the workforce and its functionality. Whilst it could be conceptualisation of any organisation's structure and may have high and low combination of various elements, systematic views of the structure have many dimensions to various units. Schine and colleagues (1971–1988) conducted a study to identify and reported these dimensions, which are shown below:

- Hierarchy dimension: this element is a relative rank of individuals working within the organisation to chart the level of roles and responsibilities they will have and thereby the power to make decisions
- Functional dimension: this discusses the differing services performed within the organisation
- Inclusion dimension: this demonstrates the flow of information and personnel to its core structure as shown in an organisational chart which can be complex to delineate

Dimensions in any organisation chart are planned and implemented using three key principles of formal relations and reporting lines, position of each employee in a group or unit, and the system designed to coordinate the first two points. These can be influenced by technology, institutional size, workforce, the work conducted by the institution, and overall aims. In the case of institutions that perform research, the variability of these influences is significant. For example, in the United Kingdom, the NHS delivers care through primary, secondary, and tertiary care services. Primary and secondary care in particular function independently of each other mostly, thereby the influence each of their structures have would vastly differ. As they provide both clinical and research services, their organisational structures will have two primary categories of employees making an organisational chart complex to show the reporting and hierarchy. These complexities and formalities can be centralised in some instances; all the research team conducting a study may have their own hierarchy and reporting structure. This is a common aspect explored by independent regulators and authorities such as the MHRA or CQC.

Variables impacting organisational structures

There are many organisational-level variables that could impact a structure that should be regarded for the purpose of evaluating, efficiency, and impact of research conducted on the organisation as well as the care provided to research. As such, key areas to consider as a 'variable' are listed below:

- Social structures: this represents flexible relations with low complexity. This type of organisation could design an organisation chart and hierarchy relatively easily. A good example with the NHS could be a research team conducting non-interventional studies. As these studies are mostly low risk, the team delivering the studies can have a more flexible approach to their work, thus minimal formality, and the wider team is closer to the leaders. In this context, duties or management can often be a mutual agreement with both direct and informal supervision methods being in place. Whilst this type of operational structure is uncommon in the NHS, many academic organisations based small–medium size research groups function in this manner.
- Functional structure: this represents complexity in terms of the work conducted in the organisation, but operationalisation of management uses a simple structure. A key feature of this type of structure is the increasing need for separation to function with specific roles and responsibilities allocation to achieve shared goals. An example of this type of structure would be a NHS organisation with teaching and research excellence status where clinical, research, and educational activities are delivered across multiple areas by a number of teams. Each of these teams will act independently as their roles and responsibilities are highly specific, but the ultimate goal is to provide high-quality clinical care directly and by way of education, training,

and research. This also means there is limited room to re-work activities, thus efficiency is a core end goal to maximise cost-effectiveness.

- Multidivisional structure: this is functional structure with an evolving approach to reduce decisions among senior management teams. This is a key structural trait for many NHS organisations in primary, secondary, and tertiary care as well as academic institutions where a single senior management team could lay out strategic objectives and remain distance from daily operations.

- Matrix structure: this is a structure comprising functional and multidivisional structures where the primary aims are to combine the efficiency, flexibility, and sensitivity based on work logic, patients, and geography. All organisations performing research work could use this form of structure where specialised functions are conducted by multiple project teams. Delegation of roles and responsibilities is a key feature within this structure across all employees.

- Hybrid structure: this is a structure that has two other structures within the organisation to combine the advantages of the two. Hybrid structures have become popular among specialised units such as clinical trial units due to the complex nature of research tasks completed.

- Network structure: this is a structure that uses rapidly changing processes with rigid and short life cycles, such as in instances where clinical trials with a short recruitment window or medical technology studies

These structural forms can be theoretical and practical. Theoretical structures are generic and abstract that can be categorised as organic and mechanistic. Variables such as technology and size influence if the theoretical structure is organic or mechanistic. Table 7.1 indicates key features of theoretical structures.

Practical structures are categorised into two groups, as indicated below (Fig. 7.1);

The five principles could manage the organisation and design the structure. The operative core demonstrates the workforce and the tasks they carry forth whilst the strategic apex represents the top management tier along with its supportive staff. The midpoint represents the middle management structure whilst the technical point groups the analysts for the organisation. The supportive point of the organisation demonstrates the workforce that carries out tasks allied to the management team activities. This is an important aspect to understand in order to evaluate the efficiency of the existing organisational structure and improve any areas required.

Table 7.1 The key features of organic and mechanistic structures.

Key features	
Organic structure	*Mechanistic structure*
Units have a minimal horizontal differentiation	Units are differentiated horizontally
High collaboration	Relations are exact
Lack of a centralised decision system	Centralised decision system
Tasks are delivered flexibly	Relations are flexible
High participation	Formal communication channels

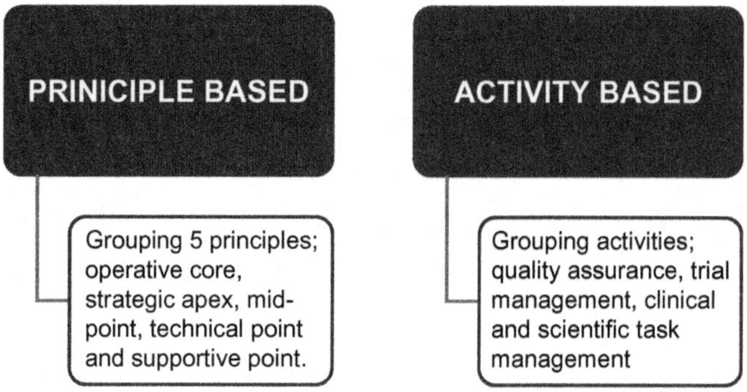

PRINICIPLE BASED

Grouping 5 principles; operative core, strategic apex, mid-point, technical point and supportive point.

ACTIVITY BASED

Grouping activities; quality assurance, trial management, clinical and scientific task management

Fig. 7.1 The two main categories which practical structures are split into.

Grouping activities is another aspect of practical structures that influences workforce interactions, including those with management and leadership teams. For example, hospitals in particular have practical structures based on activities between clinical and research tasks. This is a common premise in the United Kingdom whereby teams build a structure to ensure roles and responsibilities can be delivered, as required in each context. Some research studies require multidisciplinary professionals to be part of a treatment plan, whilst this is standard practice often clinically. For those studies that do not require multidisciplinary professionals, it can be cumbersome to keep the clinical team informed of a research protocol requirements, and vice versa. Thus, practical and theoretical premise in any type of organisation structure is complex to dissect and truly evaluate with granularity. Often, researchers use process evaluation which is a qualitative method to assess the structures from a theoretical and practical perspective, although there are many limitations to this based on real-world complexities associated within organisations.

7.2 Structure and readiness for conducting research in the United Kingdom

Organisational structure is vital to efficiently and effectively deliver the responsibilities to achieve the goals [3]. As a result of medical advancements and increasing population demands, preparedness to setup and deliver research in the United Kingdom is rapidly evolving. New structures in many organisations review team structures and their boundaries more regularly now to ensure they remain fit for purpose to deliver the research required [4,5].

Structural elements have important features, and these have evolved over the years. Bowman and Deal [6] demonstrated their opinion based on six-point hypotheses which acknowledged biases, reasoning, power, and systems aligned to the main goals. On the other hand, a four-level structural model comprising of a multilevel resource-supervision facet, alignment to laws, engagement with educational or research groups, and individual-based support including academic policies. Structural models can be prescriptive around the operational method including the various levels of duties associated with the relevant workforce [7]. The four levels are considered open, thus not hierarchical [8,9]. An example of this type of model would be small academic research groups that often have an operational framework that is vertical, with minimal or no hierarchy [10].

Primary care

Primary care research studies are set up and delivered independently in many ways. Almost two decades ago, primary care in the United Kingdom was described as a 'lost cause' [11]. Whilst this is not factually correct, often it is perceived to recruit lesser patients in comparison to research conducted in hospital environments, i.e. secondary care. Since the inception of Primary Care Research Networks (PCRNs), research in primary care has improved from a participation and study variability perspective [12,13]. The National Institute for Health Research (NIHR) portfolio demonstrates greater diversity with drug and medical device clinical trials now taking place in the primary care setting. In 2012, it was reported that 129,000 patients participated in England alone within primary care–led studies whilst 206,716 patients for those taking place in a secondary and community care setting [14].

The advantage of using primary care as a source of study participant recruitment is the vast quantity of routine data and potentially, an easier platform especially to conduct digital research studies. UK's patient registration system used by specific general practitioners is a useful method to gather longitudinal records of patients. The national identifiers allocated by way of NHS numbers enable the sharing of primary and secondary care record. This type of linked data sources are highly valuable for both data-driven research studies and promoting diversity in any research study sample. The Royal College of General Practitioners (RCGP) [15] has set up a research readiness scheme that could facilitate research in primary care. Challenges associated with multiple governance systems were one of the first features this scheme discussed to ensure that necessary training is provided to relevant staff to facilitate approvals. Since the publication of this scheme, the United Kingdom has undergone a national scale change with a single-approval-based system being implemented in the form of the Health Research Authority (HRA) which includes a single model contract that can be used to fast-track the costing and contracting procedures.

The concept of 'research readiness' has been discussed for many decades where gaps between resources available for research at any given timepoint and those dedicated to deliver research. This has significantly evolved over the COVID-19 pandemic period where primary care has played a key role in the implementation of both surveillance and vaccination research. Although, previous claims of quality improvement research assessing research concepts and its use to influence research readiness have been debated during the pandemic, many factors such as primary care health professional buy-in and time availability have been scrutinised. One factor that has supported the resourcing issues is the number of registered patients in any given GP practice which demonstrate that sharp rises in workload directly impact primary care practices ability to conduct clinical research that is required for complex conditions. For example, primary care has conducted less drug and device trials in comparison to secondary care despite the referral pathways starting from GPs. More commercial sponsors are starting to use recruitment enrichment strategies by way of including GP practices to either recruit participants at the point of diagnosis or track long-term follow-up data. The willingness to participate in research is a complex topic for most GPs due to resourcing and funding issues. One factor that could contribute to primary care being more flexible and improve their overall readiness would be to have experienced research staff directly employed to conduct more research. Whilst practices that recruit more patients are able to secure resources via the NIHR more readily, not all have the opportunity to secure these. Therefore, a more direct approach either via sponsors of these studies could be an option to consider. Primary care practices themselves could employ research staff which would be a positive investment both financially and quality improvement wise. From a financial perspective, practices would be renumerated for the research activities they deliver whilst patients would have the opportunity to take part in novel drug or medical device trials, which otherwise may not be taking place in their local hospital.

Secondary care

Research readiness dimensions

There is limited research published around the validity of conceptualised research readiness dimensions. Definitions of these dimensions remain broad although generalisability across research organisations in the United Kingdom is feasible with use of some localisation procedures. Based on these, there are four key dimensions required to continue with research readiness;

- Human resources, including workforce skills, experiences, and expertise
- Communication and engagement
- Infrastructure, including capacity and capability building of record systems, governance procedures, and business processes
- Knowledge dissemination and transfer including healthcare professional and patient readiness

Based on these dimensions, there are a large number of national policies, initiatives, and programmes put in place. These remain aligned to the UK's health and social care policy as well as framework. A large number of policies and initiatives have been in place in the United Kingdom [16], which remain aligned to the government's research and development strategy. The development and implementation of biomedical research centres, clinical trials units, and specialised research centres that design and conduct research care that may be embedded in hospitals or act as independent units are part of the UK's core research machinery. The Health and Care Act 2022 [17] demonstrates duty to conduct research and further described by the National Health Service Act 2006 that stipulates the need to facilitate research at all levels of health care services in the United Kingdom. Promotion of innovation and research has also moved forward with highly specific governance requirements implemented by the UK's Department of Health. Whilst there is much debate around the governance approaches in the United Kingdom, often described as barriers, the governance framework has been a consequence of the rapidly evolving research to meet the demands of equally complicated healthcare conditions.

The notions of human resources and infrastructure have close relationship, especially to foster a positive research culture. This is central to the success of research readiness. Some of the positive behaviours observed during the COVID-19 pandemic could be used to increase collaborations and sharing of resources and knowledge to promote good research and clinical practices. The direct notion of knowledge transfer demonstrated the use of improved evidence-based approaches being used to manage clinical care. There are risks to early evidence use in some instances, as demonstrated by fears of the use of vaccines under special circumstances during the COVID-19 pandemic. The practice of this has set a precedence to fast-track drug and medical device development which influences the human resources and infrastructural dimensions. This is further supported if reward and recognition inspire positive changes that are central to the evolution of clinical practice but also a more research-pro culture.

Whilst benchmarking various aspects of research conduct is important, fostering an appropriate assessment system that is fair, efficient, transparent, and unbiased without any disparities would further support all four dimensions. Whilst equality, equity, diversity, and inclusion are now critically discussed in comparison to previous decades, significant improvements are required to address better initiatives for patients taking part in research and the research workforce. For example, the UK's Research and Innovation (UKRI) aimed to develop and increase participation, retention, and promotion of diversely talented individuals. However, the impact of these initiatives remains to be explored and reported to understand the accountability of employers to create a more effective workforce. This has been further discussed in Chapter 10.

7.3 Structure and readiness in academia versus the NHS

Readiness in academia and the NHS have some similarities, as shown below:

- Future of clinical research is dependent upon many facets although key factors including population and disease demand, healthcare costs, research funding, healthcare system infrastructure, and availability of resources in healthcare organisations as well as higher education institutions

- Understanding, evaluating, and implementing the research landscape from a globalisation and locational perspective
- Understanding and informing the changing regulatory and legislative landscape of the United Kingdom to promote better integration of global clinical research
- Improving epidemiology research relevant to the UK population
- Improving diversity and inclusivity in clinical trials that are relevant to the UK population

---

Case study

Team structures are best formulated when barriers are eliminated where daily decisions are made by experienced operational staff working closely with the teams than centralised management teams. This concept is far more important for virtual organisations where remote working is standard practice. In such instances, the operational model and structure will also be influenced by the number of employees involved and the outcomes of the work completed. Task or goal-oriented approaches are important, and sustainability of this has a close relationship of staff engagement as well as maintenance of their well-being.

Learning objectives

- Team structures should be clear and concise. This should be documented using an organogram.
- Avoiding multiple leadership roles in a single hierarchy will promote efficiency.
- Well-being of the staff involved should be an important factor that the leader of the team should regularly review to ensure any support required can be provided promptly.
- Sustainability of performance is vital, thus preventing occupational burnout is a core responsibility of management teams. Thus, ensuring efficiency is maintained by way of using linear processes would be useful.

References

[1] Mintzberg H. The myths of MIS. Calif Manag Rev 1972;15(1):92–7. https://doi.org/10.2307/41164405.
[2] Arnold HJ, Feldman DC. Organization behavior. vol. 1; 1986. New York.
[3] Arabi M. The design of organizational structure. Tehran: Cultural Research Office; 2007.
[4] Bush T, Hamid SA, Ng A, Kaparou M. School leadership theories and the Malaysia education blueprint: findings from a systematic literature review. Int J Educ Manag 2018;32(7):1245–65.

[5] Tafreshi Q, Yusefi R, Khadivi A. A new attitude to views of organization and management. Tehran: Andishe Farashenakhti Publications; 2002.

[6] Bolman LG, Deal TE. Reframing organizations: artistry, choice, and leadership. John Wiley & Sons; 2017.

[7] Johatch M. Organization theory. Translated by Dr. H. Danayifard, Tehran: Mehban Publications; 2014.

[8] Daft R. Theory and design of organization. Translated by Parsian and Arabi, Tehran: Cultural Research Office; 1998.

[9] Rabbinz S. The basics of organizational management. Translated by Parsian and Arabi, Tehran: Cultural Research Office; 2012.

[10] Rezayian A. The basics of organization and management. Tehran: SAMT Publications; 2005.

[11] Is primary-care research a lost cause? Lancet 2003;361(9362):977.

[12] McAvoy BR. Primary care research–what in the world is going on? Med J Aust 2005;183(2):110–2.

[13] Sullivan F, Butler C, Cupples M, Kinmonth AL. Primary care research networks in the United Kingdom. BMJ 2007;334(7603):1093–4. https://doi.org/10.1136/bmj.39190.648785.80.

[14] The National Institute for Health Research (NIHR), Clinical Research Network. More patients taking part in primary care research: number of patients participating in primary care-focused research doubles over a year. Guardian 2012. 29 October http://www.theguardian.com/healthcare-network-nihr-clinical-research-zone/more-patients-primary-care-research. [Accessed 23 June 2022].

[15] Royal College of General Practitioners (RCGP). Research ready self-accreditation, http://www.rcgp.org.uk/clinical-and-research/research-opportunities-and-awards/research-ready-self-accreditation.aspx. [Accessed 23 June 2022].

[16] UK Research and Development Roadmap. The government's Research and Development (R&D) Roadmap sets out the UK's vision and ambition for science, research and innovation, https://www.gov.uk/government/publications/uk-research-andevelopment-roadmap/uk-research-and-development-roadmap. [Accessed 23 June 2022].

[17] Health and Care Act. Health service in England: integration, collaboration and other changes., 2022, https://www.legislation.gov.uk/ukpga/2022/31/contents/enacted. [Accessed 23 June 2022].

Further reading

Reitman ZJ, Paolella BR, Bergthold G, Pelton K, Becker S, Jones R, Beroukhim R. Mitogenic and progenitor gene programmes in single pilocytic astrocytoma cells. Nat Commun 2019;10(1):1–17.

8

Research capacity and capability

Key messages

- Research capacity and capability building in an ongoing process where the primary driving force is funding.
- Assessing policies, resources, and service users as part of research capacity and capability procedures undertaken in the United Kingdom is important for all external and internal sponsoring organisations.
- The National Institute for Health Research provides research capability funding (RCF) to all National Healthcare System organisation that undertake clinical research.
- Ethics committees should consider assessing capability and capacity as this is a core ethical principle to ensure suitable infrastructure is available for all participants.

8.1 Background

Capacity could be defined by the development of organisations, staff, and associated infrastructure to strengthen the capability to achieve their objectives over time. Building capacity and capability can be twofold, including human and infrastructure development.

Capacity development associated with human development focuses on expansion of human capabilities which equate to increasing the knowledge and knowledge-transfer basis in addition to promoting and empowering people to express their freedom and equality.

8.2 Professional perspectives

Healthcare professionals are fundamental for the success of clinical research, which is why the divide between clinical research and clinical practice is one of the most paramount issues

Clinical Trials and Tribulations. https://doi.org/10.1016/B978-0-12-821787-0.00004-0

that clinical research is currently facing. There is a significant lack of involvement from frontline clinicians in clinical research which reduces the number of referrals of patients to clinical trials, as well as the total number of principal investigators available to run trials. Furthermore, research that has been conducted within academic medical centres rather than within non-teaching hospitals is less likely to be uptaken with the daily practice of the hospital. It is imperative that to generate clinical research that will be implemented in clinical practice, healthcare professionals must be actively engaged throughout the clinical trial process.

If healthcare professionals are not actively involved within the clinical process and are not engaged with supporting the changes, it will have a cascade of negative impacts, resulting in a slow uptake of evidence-based interventions. For many clinical trials, the characteristics of the study participants, their comorbidities, and usual therapeutic interventions, the study setting, and the criteria for which the trial is conducted vary in resemblance to what usually occurs within a community practice, thus resulting in outcomes that have no meaning to real-world practice and therefore redundant in use. As the outcomes potentially have little impact upon clinicians' practices, it can explain why some physicians show hesitation to be involved within clinical research that aims to modify their current treatment practice to mirror the findings from the clinical trial. This separation between healthcare professionals involved in clinical trials and those who are not actively engaged in research is one of the major issues that prevent successful translation from research to real-life clinical setting. For any improvement in implementation of clinical research to be made, the divergence between the current separate entities of clinical trials and clinical practice must converge.

In oncology, it is frequently reported that only 3%–5% of eligible patients enrol in oncology clinical trials which is a clear indication that clinical research is failing to recruit an appropriate number of patients. An often cited barrier to participation within research has been the lack of familiarity with and the inability to access clinical trials shown by healthcare professionals, with an overall lack of interest for referring patients. Healthcare professionals play a pivotal role in advising, influencing, and providing guidance to patients who are eligible for participation in clinical research. Research has consistently shown that physicians and nurses are among the most trusted individuals to be a dependable source for medical information, which includes clinical trials [1–3]. A study has shown that 84% patients stated that if their clinician recommended a trial for them to participate in, they would be more inclined to enrol. This trust in physicians is shared globally as 71% of global study volunteers confirm prior to deciding to participate in a clinical trial they speak to their physician for guidance.

Research has shown that clinicians often take a more stringent, idiosyncratic approach for selecting participants who fit the eligibility criteria. It is known that some clinicians only opt for certain patients with a health status and prognosis that is even better than what is necessary by the trial protocol (REF). Clinicians' attitudes and beliefs in regard to a patient's willingness to participate, their understanding of the trials, and ability to adhere to the protocol may make them more hesitant to inform patients of trials. This presumption from clinicians about patient's willingness to enrol in trials is not warranted as Jenkins et al. [4] concluded that 83% of patients are willing to participate if given all the necessary trial information. Moreover, other clinicians may also show reluctance to enrol patients into trials if the treatment being tested may result in more potential side effects. If those that enrol in the clinical trials have an initial better health outcome compared to older and sicker patients, this will result in the trial participants having improved outcomes than would be evident if the new treatments were tested in actual clinical practices.

For many clinicians, it is the lack of infrastructure that is a barrier for their involvement in clinical trials. Ford et al. [5] conducted a survey to test clinicians' attitudes towards clinical trials for cancer therapy, which found clinicians who worked at specialist centres are more research focused than individuals in general hospitals. This finding can be understood as specialist centres often have a better infrastructure, in terms of having more staff members and additional resources necessary to conduct trials. Specialist centres often have an affiliation or are attached to research institutes, and therefore, staff may be more research-oriented. For these staff members that have a stronger research focus, it seems they are more aware of the barrier clinicians who are reluctant to enrol patients have to the success of the clinical trial. This may impact and determine the awareness that clinicians from specialist centres have surrounding clinical trials needs. The barriers clinicians hold that prevent the success of clinical trials are then more likely to be addressed.

There is a widespread concern that research may negatively alter the doctor–patient relationship, as a patient's participation in research or a clinical trial may damage their rapport with their physician. This rapport may further be exacerbated if clinicians do not have a comprehensive grasp of what the trial entails, creating a perceived internal conflict between clinicians and their patients. Following on, there are a multitude of other challenges that could prevent healthcare professionals engaging in clinical research. Continuously busy clinical practices make for an over-burdened workload, resulting in limited opportunity for involvement in clinical trials. This results in a lack of time for healthcare professionals to gather and analyse clinical trial information and have the necessary time to discuss with eligible patients the possibility of enrolment. A questionnaire completed by physicians and nurses who were actively involved in a clinical trial concluded several centre-related barriers that hinder the success of the trial. The responses recorded that 72% of healthcare professionals view lack of available time and resources that are specific to research within the clinic. Additionally, the lack of appropriate human resources to conduct clinical trials, such as research nurses, is also an important factor for conducting clinical research, with 31% of respondents agreeing.

However, there may be some benefit for frontline clinicians to be involved within research as there is a widely held assumption that an improved healthcare performance is witnessed when engagement in research is evident by frontline healthcare professionals and organisations. The review by Boaz et al. [6] of 21 'by-product' papers suggested that clinicians and healthcare professionals who engage within research show an increased likelihood of improvement in healthcare performance. As there is a need to justify expenditure on research in NHS organisations, this topic of improved healthcare performance should be at the forefront for reasons why it is paramount for healthcare professionals to be involved within clinical research.

A further barrier is the current lack of support within the clinical research infrastructure, especially with limited administrative assistance and financial support. Financial incentives for healthcare professionals is one method to encourage physicians to recruit for clinical trials. This type of incentive is what some UK research funders, especially the pharmaceutical industry, do to entice healthcare professionals to recruit patients. This method of incentivising is used but is rare within publicly funded trials. For example, the NHS HTA programme, a publicly funded research programme, would have to provide a considerable amount of evidence to suffice paying monetary incentives to be considered a viable method. A substantial number of clinical trials within the NHS rely on the academic interest and goodwill of the healthcare professionals with alternative incentives such as recognition of involvement in the trial through authorship.

Following on, the United Kingdom is one of the most prestigious nations across the globe to undertake research in the life sciences industry. The Life Sciences Industry is a major contributor to the UK economy, contributing over £70 billion per year and employment to 240,000 individuals. The strategy utilises the established strengths of research conducted in the United Kingdom: the capability in clinical and translational medicine in the NHS; a highly skilled workforce; establishing the usage of emerging fields within life science industry, such as artificial intelligence (AI) and the move to a more digitalised healthcare. The strategy sets to establish novel industries within the fields of early detection of disease and the advancement of technologies and therapies. Moreover, the strategy acknowledges there are areas within this industry that have resulted in a reduced growth; for example, the slow uptake of novel technologies; the barriers to successfully scale up biotech companies and to continue the drive for Research and Development Departments to receive funding that will enable the production of globally competitive research.

This strategy call from the life science industry resulted in a response from the government to create a first Life Sciences Sector Deal. The deal included an investment over £1 billion for innovative investment in the industry and close to £500 million for the life science industry to support research programmes. In 2018, a second Life Sciences Sector Deal was created to produce additional measures to enable the United Kingdom to become global leads in specific areas within the life science industry. These deals will enable the industry to accelerate and provide the most innovative diagnostics, therapies, medicines, and digital platforms. By creating these opportunities, it provides benefits for both grow within the UK economy and creating this growth for a sustainable NHS.

8.3   Roles in clinical research

Conducting clinical research is probably the ultimate in team working. The core team that is directly involved in the research includes the chief investigator (CI), principal investigator (PI), co-investigators, research practitioners, and study co-ordinators. This team must work with other staff who may not be directly involved in the research. They may include clinical staff, specialist nurses, pharmacists, and other support staff.

The team involved should be aware of the individual and collective roles and it is for the PI to ensure that the delegated tasks are appropriate. International conference of Harmonisation Good Clinical Practice (GCP) guidelines defines the roles of the investigator and the research team. For example, the investigator is responsible for the health and welfare of the research subject and be aware of the research protocol and regulations. The lead investigator for each site is the PI, and the other investigators are co-investigators. The responsibility of the sponsor is taking the lead in initiating the research, as well as managing and financing it. These roles can be delegated by the sponsor. There should be a clear documentation of the roles as a part of setting up a study. While the duties can be delegated to suitably qualified members, the responsibilities are not reflected in the same sense in terms of change to job titles, in most instances.

The PI can delegate the duties to the co-investigators, research practitioners, data managers, and the clinical trial staff. For example, the screening of the patients, consenting, randomisation, and completion of case report forms can be delegated to the co-investigators and research practitioners. Data managers can be tasked with data entry and support monitoring, audits, and inspections. Table 8.1 indicates an overview of common research roles and responsibilities in place within organisations.

Table 8.1 Common roles and responsibilities with research teams.

Roles	Similar roles	Responsibilities	Type of research conducted
Chief Investigator			Epidemiology studies/ Clinical trials
Principal Investigator			All research studies
Research Project manager	Trial manager		All research studies
Clinical Trial Practitioner	Research Practitioner		All research studies
Clinical Trial Administrator	Research Administrator		Clinical trials
Research Nurse	Clinical Research Nurse		All research studies
Clinical Research Fellow	Research Fellow		All research studies
Epidemiologist	Clinical Epidemiologist		Epidemiology studies
Research Associate	Post-doctoral researcher		All research studies
Research Assistant	Research coordinator		All research studies
Researcher	Senior Research Fellow		All research studies
Physician Associate	N.A.		All research studies
Research scientist	Clinical Research Scientist		All research studies
Data Scientist	Data Analyst		Epidemiology studies
Clinical Trial manager	Senior Trial Manager		Clinical trials
Data Manager	N.A		Clinical trials
Data administrator	Database coordinator		Clinical trials
Research Operations Manager	Operations Manager		All research studies
Database Manager	Database Administrator		All research studies

Job descriptions and titles

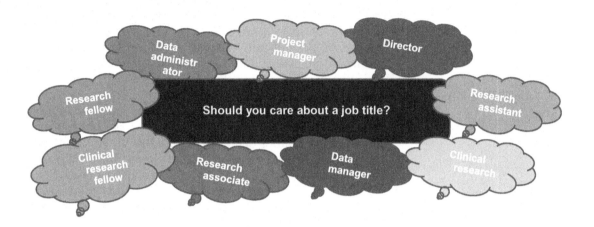

A long-standing debate has been around the use of non-standardised job descriptions and job titles. There are limitations for standardising all job descriptions pertaining to a role, although a core set of roles and responsibilities should be considered at least at an organisation level. Often, an employee's role is not justifiably demonstrated in their daily tasks. For example, some clinical trial manager job descriptions indicate the requirement to input into publications and grants when this is a specific role of a researcher. Some organisations use two job titles to ensure that the role an employee carries forth is representative, and therefore, a value-based model can be created to also retain staff for longer.

Remodelling job [7] descriptions that is more suited for the digital age is another facet to consider given that many conventional job titles are out of date in the context of a workplace where hierarchies and responsibilities have become more superfluous. Technological transformation has led to a higher pace at which new skills are acquired that boost a team and organisation's overall productivity. This also means automation of various tasks that may have been conducted manually provides further reasons to amend job titles as required to fit into new research business models. A few common examples where job titles should be reconsidered are as follows:

1. Project manager: Often this term is adapted in job descriptions as *Research Project Manager, Senior Project Manager,* or *Project Manager.* There are various perceptions and assumptions

surrounding this job title. The most common perception is that a project manager role is administrative and is not a research role. Yet a closer look at the daily working or even tasks completed throughout a period covered within an appraisal year demonstrates that a large number of tasks are researcher-based than administrative. Some academic institutions have distinctive job descriptions for these post holders whilst others have significant variations. For example, the NHS would adopt a more administrative approach when hiring a project manager while an academic organisation may take a more fluid approach with more research activities being delivered. Pay grades equally differ significantly among project managers between the NHS, academia, and industry, despite having similar roles and responsibilities. Whilst it could be argued that industry would pay more than public institutions, there should be conformity at some level to provide parity to employees who are in this role.

2. Senior Trial Manager: Senior Trial Managers (STM) have a varied job descriptions in the United Kingdom. The UK Trial Manager Network (UK-TMN) has often discussed this issue extensively, partly because of perceptions and the lack of recognition provided. As a result of this, the turnover of STMs is high in most organisations. The lack of long-term funding is another issue, especially within academic organisations where a rate-limiting factor could be limited funding available as STMs are often linked to a specific grant. Thus, securing bridge funding till another grant is secured isn't always feasible. There are more advantages of transferring an STM from a single study or a group of studies to another is more useful than hiring new staff to create a value-based model as part of staff retention and to transfer experience to more junior staff. Pay grades across STMs vary between academia, industry, and the NHS despite similar roles and responsibilities. This is another facet UK-TMN members have vocalised, in addition to having access to equal opportunities for career advancement.

3. Research coordinator: Research coordinators have flexible tasks and often non-specific to research studies. The variability in pay grades among employees with this job title between the NHS and academia is substantially different. Educational qualifications for research coordinators vastly differ, hence often these post holders are perceived as junior members of a research team.

There are advantages and disadvantages for becoming a fluid and collaborative team versus a more structured team depending on the type of clinical research conducted. The need to have transparent roles and responsibilities is unequivocally important when conducting clinical research, as demonstrated by Good Clinical Practice (GCP). However, job titles draw unnecessary boundaries for those completing duties of senior positions and could undermine high-performing employees. From a pragmatic and less conceptual standpoint, digital transformation is growing globally through various accelerated programmes, making most job descriptions and job titles obsolete.

Job titles in a job application could be perceived as an advantage or a disadvantage, depending on the perceptions as well as knowledge base around research workforce associated with the hiring manager. For example, a previous job title that is perceived as a more junior role could mean the upward progression a candidate is expecting may be prevented even before an opportunity is given to them for an interview. For candidates deciding to make a lateral move or change in career, the job title may further hamper their chances of securing a role of their choice, thereby reducing equal opportunities available to them. In addition, job titles also matter to colleagues in some cases and may even prevent collaborations from taking place if it is felt there is a lack of political leverage. For example, valuable collaborations may be declined, thereby reducing the potential to secure grants.

Job titles could often indicate position and authority, especially within the context of leadership. Traditional career pathways in research often separates those that conducted research from those managing and leading them. Supervisory roles were often held by professors. This is still the case in many organisations, although this culture is shifting to make room for more progressive ways to include those with multifaceted skills and experiences. This further impacts pay scales.

Developing research roles for the future should focus on skills rather than tasks, identifying talented individuals who could excel with transferrable skills. The *boxed-in* roles that have historically existed, where employees would only deliver a set number of tasks, need to change. Emphasising the need for people development and growth should be a key principle that should remain the focus on recruitment managers. It is important to build skill maps and core competency maps as well as responsibilities at individual and team level to allow flexibility as well as knowledge scaffolds to ensure performance is sustained short, medium, to long-term. Employees should be empowered especially within high-pressure settings where study protocols demand stringent working methods and rapid adaptability.

Job specifications and skill maps

Job specifications in research require adaptability from a broader sense especially for those working in clinical trials and epidemiology studies where the requirements to successfully report the outcomes need flexibility. Thus, recommended or essential qualities along with desirable features should be considered in an adaptable manner. The knowledge summary of a job specification can often act as a catalyst for interview panels to decide the suitability of a candidate, which can sometimes remove perfectly good candidates from securing a position. Thus, there are advantages and disadvantages of using job specifications. Whilst it is advantageous to highlight job specifications to employees and HR managers, the threshold framework could also be used during performance appraisals and considerations for benchmarking performance. Writing a specification, especially if these are non-standardised, writing these can be time-consuming for hiring managers which is a disadvantage especially in large teams and departments. The use of a threshold framework could also be a disadvantage as emotional intelligence and personality traits cannot be assessed using this method. Even if personality tests were used as part of understanding a potential employee, forecasting behaviours would be challenging.

To address challenges with job specifications, a skill map with a core competency map could be used. The candidate and the recruitment manager could complete this to ensure a transparent and fare recruitment process could be completed. Fig. 8.1 shows a useful set of skills to consider when building a skill map that can be used for all research posts with various adjustments that demonstrated in Fig. 8.1.

The skill map can be an evolving document that covers an array of skills that a candidate or employee has in addition to those acquired. The skill maps can be kept linear and adaptable to any role to ensure recruitment managers as well as line managers are able to complete these efficiently.

Communication competency should be an integral part of a skill map, in particular for managerial and leadership roles. Behavioural dimensions are fundamental to setting a professional and positive working culture. This has a direct and an indirect relationship with staff retention and organisational reputation. Key components of behavioural dimensions required for communication competency are shown in Fig. 8.2.

Behavioural dimensions are complex, thus underlying team dynamics could attribute to workplace culture, communication, and the overall skill map. A large number of quality improvement and behavioural intervention-associated research studies have

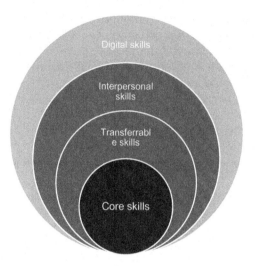

Fig. 8.1 A theme of skills that can be used when employing research staff. This can act as a competency framework that can combine core, technical, and behavioural skills required to deliver a job requirement. This could replace a job specification. Alternatively, this can also be used as part of probationary meetings and appraisals.

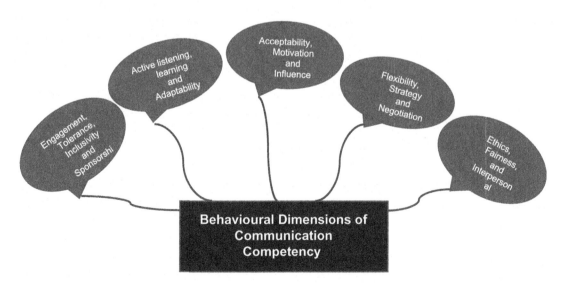

Fig. 8.2 Key components of behavioural dimensions of communication competency.

been conducted to develop competency frameworks and influence change with a view to improve employee relations. However, most of these behavioural interventions have not been adopted in workplaces. In research environments, whilst hospital and academic settings in particular may have differences, the ethos of conducting and delivering research remains the same. Thus, skill maps could be a better method to have ongoing evaluations and discussions around behaviour to influence change where it is needed.

Case study

Core competencies and skills are fundamental to developing a comprehensive job description. The extent of the core skills and competencies vary based on the experience level required to successfully deliver the role. The competencies could also vary by the type of education and training completed by a candidate. There is a list of informatic domains with specialist concepts that should be considered, as shown below:

- Medical informatics
- Clinical informatics
- Pharmacy informatics
- Nursing informatics
- Clinical bioinformatics
- Public health informatics
- Social-care informatics
- Health data science

Researchers have provided evidence and iterative approaches to analyse complexities around competency definitions and the association of these included within a job description. For example, commonality among informatics disciplines is important to understand the overarching skills that could aid with appointing candidates that have transferrable skills. Perfectly good candidates are eliminated especially within academia if direct skills are not available. Therefore, understanding subdisciplines and building these into job descriptions is a helpful approach to consider. Paucity of health informaticians and/or analysts that understand healthcare data in the United Kingdom is a wider problem, and training those who may not have direct skills could be a better way to fill a position than maintain under-resourced teams.

The use of validated competency frameworks and skill maps is important as domain knowledge advancement and knowledge management should be considered. Common competencies and skills used to develop frameworks and skills are demonstrated in the below figure below [2,3,8]. Using Fig. 8.3, roles can be standardised which will aid with sharing skills across disciplines. Broader competencies and accreditations from professional societies should be considered as method to assess experience levels to assess salary scales and to put forward developmental plans.

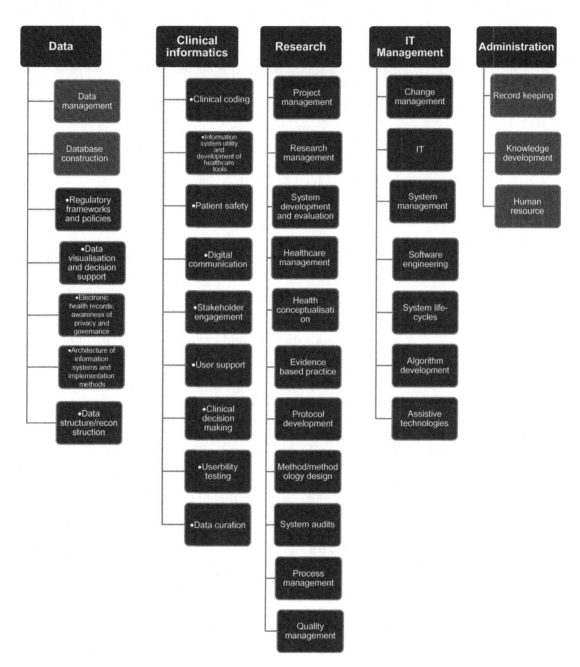

Fig. 8.3 The various roles within clinical research teams.

Learning outcomes

Learning outcomes of developing suitable job roles with appropriate specifications are an important part of managing research operations and sustaining high-quality operational outputs. Following recommendations that could be considered by human resource departments and hiring managers:

- The use of suitable job titles that reflect the work completed by a post-holder is a good first point. Ensuring any changes to the job are equally reflected with the job title should be considered and implemented where possible
- Simple economy-to-scale approaches should be used with the help of graduate entry programmes to utilise diverse backgrounds
- Develop exchange programmes for doctoral and/or medical students to obtain skills in clinical informatics could assist manage paucity of resources medium to long-term
- Better educational programmes should be considered to promote informatics education with the use of introducing these in an array of sciences
- Robust evaluations should be used to assess performance of staff and provide ongoing training to help build capacity
- Opportunities to grow within the roles and development of new roles should be considered
- Provide variation in working environments, and flexibility to ensure professional growth is supported
- Flexibility with competency, training, and curriculum development should be reflected where cross-cutting informatics knowledge remains as a primary focus
- Developing leadership/management roles with system development and evaluation should be considered

References

[1] Greenhalgh T, Macfarlane F. Towards a competency grid for evidence-based practice. J Eval Clin Pract 1997;3:161–5. https://doi.org/10.1046/j.1365-2753.1997.00082.x.

[2] Delanerolle G, Zeng Y, Phiri P, Phan T, Tempest N, Busuulwa P, et al. Systematic review and meta-analysis of mental health impact on BAME populations with preterm birth. medRxiv 2022. https://doi.org/10.1101/2022.03.22.22272780.

[3] Delanerolle G, Thayanandan T, Riga J, Griffiths J, Lawson J, Au-Yeung S, et al. Clinical trials: from problem child to the driving force of medical advancement. Br J Neurosci Nurs 2020;16(5). https://doi.org/10.12968/bjnn.2020.16.5.200.

[4] Jenkins JM, Caldwell DA, Chandrasekaran H, Twicken JD, Bryson ST, Quintana EV, Clarke BD, Li J, Allen CD, Tenenbaum P, Wu H, Klaus TC, Middour CK, Cote MT, McCauliff S, Girouard FR, Gunter JP, Wohler B, Sommers J, Hall JR, Uddin K, Wu MS, Bhavsar PA, Cleve JE, Pletcher DL, Dotson J, Haas MR, Gilliland RL,

Koch DG, Borucki WJ. Overview of the Kepler science processing pipeline. Astrophys J 2010;713:87.

[5] Foy R, Parry J, Duggan A, Delaney B, Wilson S, Lewin-Van Den Broek NT, Lassen A, Vickers L, Myres P. How evidence based are recruitment strategies to randomized controlled trials in primary care? Experience from seven studies. Family Pract 2003;2003(20):83–92.

[6] Boaz A, Hanney S, Jones T, et al. Does the engagement of clinicians and organisations in research improve healthcare performance: a three-stage review. BMJ Open 2015;5, e009415. https://doi.org/10.1136/bmjopen-2015-009415.

[7] Smith T. It's time to rethink job descriptions for the digital era. Available from: https://hbr.org/2021/12/its-time-to-rethink-job-descriptions-for-the-digital-era.

[8] Delanerolle G. The triple E: equality, equitable health care, and empowerment – are we there yet? Br J Gen Pract 2022;72(717):150–1. https://doi.org/10.3399/bjgp22X718841.

Further reading

Breil B, Kremer L, Taweel A, Lux T. A comparative literature analysis of the health informatics curricula. Proc IEEE/ACS Int Conf Comput Syst Appl AICCSA 2018;2019:1–4. https://doi.org/10.1109/AICCSA.2018.8612821.

Gardner RM, Overhage JM, Steen EB, Munger BS, Holmes JH, Williamson JJ, et al. Core content for the subspecialty of clinical informatics. J Am Med Informatics Assoc 2009;16:153–7. https://doi.org/10.1197/jamia.M3045.

9

Research waste

Key messages

- Research waste occurrs at every level of the research development and conduct process. As a result, publications would undoubtedly attribute to research waste.
- Inconsistencies in research studies and their interpretations add confusion to the body of evidence available, therefore add to the generation of research waste.
- Unreliable information further complicates problems with research waste.
- Repurposing method and practices should be considered to better manage research waste.
- Prescription medicine waste is a global epidemic. This causes an estimated annual loss of £300 million in the United Kingdom alone.

9.1   Background [1–6]

Research waste is a well-established concept in clinical research and can be defined by a broad description although the general consensus is that it is the product of research outcomes that lack patient and societal benefit and has multifactorial causes. Knowledge generation, translation of this to clinical practice, and its suitability are important features to consider throughout the research process from the design of the research question, methods, patient acceptance and service accessibility, to the real-world applicability and implementation to healthcare systems. In 2009, research waste was estimated to amount to a total of US$ 85 billion.

Research waste could be categorised into basic and clinical research. Basic research could include translational and pre-clinical research. Clinical research refers to applied and bio-medical research. The use of these different categories and sub-categories is not as previously thought of as a generation of new knowledge and impactful evidence has developed. The cost of these different categories varies globally. For example, the global investment in biomedical research has increased year on year and both patients and researchers are the principal beneficiaries. In the United Kingdom, over £1.6 billion in research investment was made between 2009 and 2010 alone, whereas a similar pattern was demonstrated in the USA in 2012. The assertion of such investments needs to be reviewed against subsequent clinical advances and overall improvements made within healthcare systems. The pathway for development of research in general is convoluted and is influenced by the clinical specialty and whether the work is exploratory or not. For example, research conducted to explore drugs in comparison to complex interventions will have different developmental pathways as discussed in Chapter 1. Basic sciences underpin clinical research, thus, if accurate, they are adaptable and translatable to various clinical research areas.

A key method to quantify research waste would be to conduct a cumulative meta-analysis to demonstrate the current evidence and effectiveness of the interventions in current practice over a period of time, effect size, and as a result, any gaps identified. Stable or precise effect sizes provide valuable insight from a comprehensively conducted meta-analysis. There are a number of novel methods that have further developed the field of meta-analyses which can act as a double-edged sword in some areas of medicine where a high heterogeneity is observed due to the nature of the complex conditions, such as multimorbidity or disease sequalae.

9.2 Addressing research waste

Research waste should be addressed as a priority. Organisations conducting research, funders, and industry alike should be responsible and accountable for ensuring high-quality research that is relevant to patients directly and indirectly is delivered. Whilst it is vital to acknowledge researchers' interest in influencing research studies, a strong sense of patients as priorities need to remain in place as the focal point during the developmental stages. For this reason, research proposals from senior researchers are more likely to receive approval for funding, as opposed to those from less experienced members of staff. However, whilst experience plays a vital role when conducting research, this means that novel ideas can remain unfunded even though they may be valuable to patients, if the primary researcher is perceived to be inexperienced. Additionally, although professional reputation and trustworthiness add value to research, these elements could also introduce unconscious biases and perceptions that can limit the funding of good studies that are led by early to mid-career researchers. This is an aspect of research waste that can be easily prevented through transparent peer reviews, the introduction of pragmatic and equal opportunities that can be evaluated at the beginning and end of an award period, and better evaluation reporting to funders and regulators.

Research waste also carries ethical issues surrounding the study design, data accessibility and usability in particular. A weak study design could result in cumulative waste of resources, time, and costs. A common example is the completion of pilot studies that are underpowered. Most research ethics committees and funders agree on conducting pilot studies with smaller sample sizes due to a variety of reasons, including risks pertaining to cost-efficiency if the study fails (which is commonly observed in complex intervention studies conducted in primary care and drug trials with minimal pre-clinical data associated with adverse events). Funders and regulators should have flexible approaches when funding pilot studies as novel methods, including '*start and stop*' approaches incorporated in a study design. Taking more novel and flexible approaches to sample size adjustments, including statistical simulation, could resolve underpower issues.

Historically, primary and secondary care research has been conducted separately for a variety of reasons. However, a more joined-up method of working may not only benefit patients and improve cost pressures, but could also reduce the research waste that is often observed. Unified studies with multiple work streams could provide improved primary and secondary care research outcomes as well as better use of existing resources (e.g. multi-morbidity research). This could also lead to the completion of research in shorter timeframes in some instances. There are many other ways to reduce research waste throughout the research life cycle, as shown below:

- Improving efficiency throughout the process of research study setup and conduct
- Increasing research value through priority setting
- Increasing research outputs by way of efficient study design
- Optimising the use of gathered data
- Better use of routine clinical data to better evaluate clinical needs
- Improved methods of research implementation and dissemination
- Using multiple patient recruitment settings, such as both primary and secondary care when delivering research studies
- Building cost-effective evaluations for proposed interventions from early phases
- Use of linear mechanisms and processes

- Improving funding allocations for pre-clinical and clinical studies with more research programme funds to ensure continuity of research studies
- Inclusive approaches in terms of resource use and availability of better employment contracts
- Availability of job opportunities for mid-career researchers
- Developing better methods to use clinical and research data
- Efficient use of infrastructure
- Better open science approaches and ensuring novel research ideas are fostered by journal editors
- Alignment of policies, processes, and understanding of research conduct between funders, regulators, and researchers
- Use of patient and site recruitment enrichment strategies
- Use of flexible and diverse approaches for long-term follow-up of participants to improve patient retention and longitudinal data collection
- Improving evidence synthesis methods and basic science research

Case study

Key point:

A case definition is vital and, in some instances, promotes selection bias. This is particularly important in the case of Sudden Infant Death Syndrome (SIDS) that has incurred on a bed with another person where accidental suffocation is used as an external risk factor. An improved selection bias could have been reported in publications if all SIDS cases included a post-mortem finding. In addition, a standardised definition for sleep positions should have been used as parental and resulting clinical reports differed. The most common definition of infant sleeping position was 'position place last sleep'.

Sudden and Unexpected Infant Death (SUID) or SIDS was identified as a key factor of mortality in the United Kingdom and USA during the 20th century. During the 1940s, most infant deaths were explored through autopsies where pathologist suggested this could be due to maternal overlying and accidental mechanical suffocation. In 1944, a pathologist from New York stipulated the cause of death of two-thirds of infants may be due to mechanical suffocation and face down as oppose to the common sleeping position. This evidence was corroborated by reports from the United Kingdom and Australia which led to a campaign that recommended parents to avoid sleeping on their front. In 1945, a paediatrician rejected this hypothesis and proposed that oxygen deprivation due to layers of blankets obstructed their breathing. Alternative hypotheses published included immune response or a hypersensitive reaction to inhaled milk, an undetermined infection, and inhaled vomit which dented the hypothesis of sleeping position.

However, the first case–control studies were not published until 1956 and 1958, in the USA and the United Kingdom, respectively [7]. The strength of the evidence associated with SIDS was reviewed at various time points, although a key meta-analysis performed by Ruth Gilbert and colleagues demonstrated the fundamental flaws of using practices with minimal evidence. The systematic review and meta-analysis performed by Gilbert and colleagues covered 1940–2002. The pooled evidence by 1970 indicated that two studies demonstrated that the risk of SIDS [8] was statistically high among babies sleeping on the front than back. In addition, harmful effects of infants sleeping on the back were lowest in the presence of a higher prevalence of infants sleeping in the front position. There was evidence that demonstrated sleeping in the front position elevated motor development, pylori stenosis, longer sleep duration, and nappy rash potentially due to reduced physiological control of autonomic, respiratory, and cardiovascular mechanisms.

Learning outcomes

1. Delayed recognition of the risks of front sleeping was due to the paucity of robustly conducted studies between 1970 and 1986.
2. Study designs presented issues where heterogeneity and statistical methods accurately assess these facets were not explored.
3. Another study design issue was around grouping methods used, where most lacked a comparator.
4. The relationship between the prevalence of front sleeping, time frame, and odds ratios was poor.
5. Earlier recognition of the risk associated with front sleeping could have prevented >60,000 infant deaths.
6. Use of accumulated evidence from randomised controlled trials could have been used along with observational studies. This combined approach using systematic review and meta-analysis could have highlighted effective treatments and its interpretation could have reduced spurious precision, healthy-adopter phenomenon and bias.
7. Continuous improvements to study designs as well as retrospective synthesis of the evidence through the use of comprehensive systematic reviews and meta-analyses should be common practice. This was not so in the 1970s, making it challenging for professionals and policy-makers alike to assess cumulative effects. However, the data should have been used to promote evidence-based practices that would have emphasised an earlier publication to change practice.
8. An effective case definition is a fundamental requirement as this could prevent subsequent definitions being proposed. Adapting or amending an existing definition is a better way to conduct a research study, so as to a standardised approach could be used to cvaluate any endpoints in using evidence-based approaches. This in turn would prevent research waste.

References

[1] Grainger MJ, Bolam FC, Stewart GB, Nilsen EB. Evidence synthesis for tackling research waste. Nat Ecol Evol 2020;4:495–7. https://doi.org/10.1038/s41559-020-1141-6.

[2] Glasziou P, Chalmers I. Research waste is still a scandal—an essay by Paul Glasziou and Iain Chalmers. BMJ 2018;363:k4645. https://doi.org/10.1136/bmj.k4645.

[3] Chalmers I, Glasziou P. Avoidable waste in the production and reporting of research evidence. Lancet 2009;374(9683):86–9. https://doi.org/10.1016/s0140-6736(09)60329-9.

[4] Fraser H, Parker T, Nakagawa S, Barnett A, Fidler F. Questionable research practices in ecology and evolution. PLoS ONE 2018;13, e0200303. https://doi.org/10.1371/journal.pone.0200303.

[5] Nilsen EB, Bowler D, Linnell JDC. Exploratory and confirmatory research in the open science era. J Appl Ecol 2020. https://doi.org/10.1111/1365-2664.13571.

[6] Gurevitch J, Koricheva J, Nakagawa S, Stewart G. Meta-analysis and the science of research synthesis. Nature 2018;555:175–82. https://doi.org/10.1038/nature25753.

[7] Boaz A, Hanney S, Jones T, et al. Does the engagement of clinicians and organisations in research improve healthcare performance: a three-stage review. BMJ Open 2015;5, e009415. https://doi.org/10.1136/bmjopen-2015-009415.

[8] Goldberg N, Rodriguez-Prado Y, Tillery R, Chua C. Sudden infant death syndrome: a review. Pediatr Ann 2018;47(3):e118–23. https://doi.org/10.3928/19382359-20180221-03.

10

Research operations management

Key messages
- Research operations management principles are based on operation research.
- Operational research is a combination of scientific concepts, empirical evidence generated through experience and analytical methods to problem solve and improve the decision-making processes.
- Basic concepts of research operations management in the United Kingdom differ to other parts of the world as they are based on the premise of the National Healthcare System.
- The use of four key theories of business process design, configurable system mapping, evidence-based decision-making, and continuous improvement with sustainable approaches is important for research operations management.

10.1 Background

Research operations management defines the characterisation, orchestration, and optimisation of research staff with regards to setup, management and delivery of clinical trials using processes to amplify the efficiency, value, and impact of research. A large proportion of research operations focus on research practices and the collective efforts of research staff and participants taking part in the study. Often research operations will focus on a specific framework comprising of planning, conducting, and closure (Fig. 10.1). These categories could be further sub-classified when there are multiple studies within a research project.

(a) Fig. 10.1 shows that research operations management features could be classified based on clinical research type. Research projects could house a number of different facets from a mixture of pre-clinical and clinical studies embedded with key objectives and endpoints to be delivered to answer a broader research question. Clinical trials and observational studies

Clinical Trials and Tribulations. https://doi.org/10.1016/B978-0-12-821787-0.00014-3

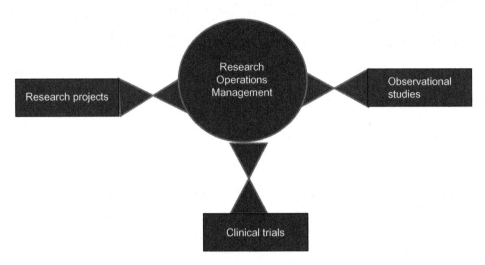

Fig. 10.1 The features of the research operations management.

equally require different research operations management strategies and methods, especially in comparison to research projects that would require long-term management goals.

(b) Fig. 10.2 demonstrates key feature of research operations management associated within all the classifications associated with a research project.

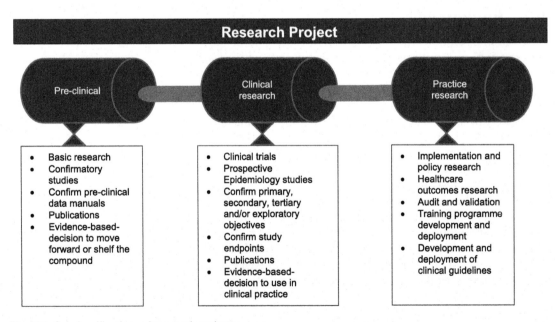

Fig. 10.2 Subclassifications of research projects.

Management theories for clinical research

Management in clinical research can be defined as a process that influences the efforts of others to achieve aims within a structured organisational setting with prescribed roles. Management theories in healthcare are crucial for developing optimal management of clinical research. The knowledge base for research management should have a strong front-line local micro-system that aligns with the UK's healthcare system expectations and Health and Social Care framework. The nature of the knowledge required to manage clinical research is proliferated by factors such as strategies, operational framework, fragmentation of information, and context dependency, to coordinate the actions required to setup, conduct, and deliver research. The public and private sectors use different research management methods based on differing performance targets, multi-stakeholder requirements, ethical implications, and values that are imperative to uphold good practices leading to high-quality research outputs. The complexities, diverse boundaries, and mechanisms lead to varying processes that could be used for optimal research management. This collective information has led to a variety of management theories that are based on a number of categories, as shown in Table 10.1.

Promoting effective and efficient work processes to develop knowledge management and other attributes helps develop a multi-skilled research team that is able to deliver research objectives. Individual assessments to develop value-based models could assist with managing and sharing knowledge within research teams aiding to recognise and value contributions made by staff. This could aid in improving professional relationships and staff retention, which would further help with advancing innovation.

Situational leadership theory

Situational leadership theory is a good concept to use when leading and developing research teams as it uses an adaptive leadership approach in which the core aspect is about encouraging staff to expand on their skills. This style of leadership is highly flexible and easily adapts to the needs of different studies and work environments. Within research, this theory can be furthered by modifying the style to include management as well given that research studies require a significant level of oversight, as recommended by regulators and sponsoring governing bodies. Thus, the adaptability component of this leadership style is suitable for a

Table 10.1 Various elements of management within clinical research.

Category	Key features	Source information
Research culture	Transparency, professional trust, professional courtesy, professional respect, and support	Open communication and mutual respect in a team strengthen relationships and enable to reach common goals in a unified manner. This type of culture promotes a positive and supportive environment that makes employees feel valued and helps maintain optimal performance by way of improved staff retention periods.
Research leadership	Shared vision and goals, effective policies and communication, effective and dependable structure, efficient managerial processes and attributes, development of strategic aims, and promoting change management	Effective leaders are able to remain competitive and relevant, maintaining incremental increases and securing funds to develop the team. Development of team dynamics is a vital.
Knowledge management	Encouraging innovation, developing expertise, strong leadership, and management to grow the team	
Research strategy	Developing a pro-research culture, role recognition, acquisition of new knowledge, talent management, information dissemination in a transparent way, value staff, and internal management of staff growth, promoting knowledge transfer, support teamwork, setting a culture of equality, and the use of change management to promote external contacts	
Human resources	Developing flexible working schemes, providing appraisals, multi-skill job specification development, and promoting positive learning–working cultures	

rapidly changing research landscape where innovations set new research paradigms required to develop research and understand unmet clinical needs. There are two models of situational leadership, one theory developed by Daniel Goleman and the other by Ken Blanchard and Paul Hershey. Daniel Goleman's theory is more widely used as many related to his book *Emotional Intelligence*, which describes six approached to leadership, as shown below:

- Coaching leaders: these leaders focus on professional and personal development ensuring employees remain content. This approach improves performance and retention of staff. Research indicates that this approach is suitable for people that are accepting of change.
- Democratic leaders: this approach gives all staff the right to vocalise their opinion in all decisions made within a team. This can improve flexibility and an ethos of self-responsibility. However, a limitation is that this approach is time-consuming and hence, not suitable for a team with multifaceted research that has multiple deadlines.
- Pace-setting leaders: these leaders promote high expectations from all their staff and are suitable for driven, highly motivated and ambitious individuals. This approach focuses on providing a great deal of flexibility to employees as it aligns with their personal beliefs and work ethic. A limitation of this is that it could lead to burn-out for the leader and employees if it is not implemented within caution.
- Affiliative leaders: employees are the primary focus with this approach where the team morale is low. Using praise and supportive strategies could assist with rebuilding confidence among with the team. A significant limitation with this approach is the risk of poor performance. Thus, using this approach along with other management strategies would be a better way to harmonise the workforce.
- Coercive leaders: focus on viewing staff as subordinates and micromanaging them, instructing each task and overseeing the work daily. This approach is useful if the organisation or team performance is poor or they have a smaller volume of research studies within a portfolio. A limitation in this approach is the high burn-out among experienced staff leading to poor retention.
- Authoritative leaders: focuses on an '*analytical problem-based approach*' to identify challenges. By employing this approach, leaders encourage their teams to be part of the conversation to resolve problems, where possible. A limitation to this approach is that it could be perceived to be more autocratic.

Employees undergo differing stages of development and alignment of these to situational leadership qualities, which could help people change from low to high competence and vice versa. This is an important component of managing research effectively, especially in the context of ensuring study protocol adherence and accurate reflection of the study objectives. Thus, situational leadership theory is relevant to clinical research leadership and

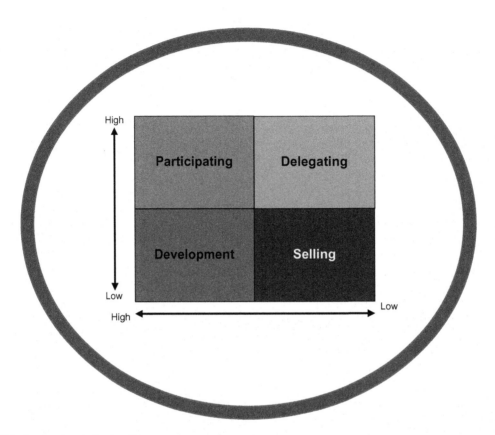

Fig. 10.3 Approaches to leadership.

management and the adaptable approaches make it favourable to deliver complex tasks (Fig. 10.3).

Situational leadership is an interesting facet to consider in research management in particular. Blanchard and colleagues theorised [1] situational leadership to be an adaptive and flexible form where a person adapts to suit the needs of their team and working environment. In order to achieve this, the leader must have acquired skills that allow them to adjust to the requirements of their team. These skills include being adaptable and flexible as they must be able to regularly assess their team's efforts and performance to ensure they are leading in the most appropriate way. This style of management is quite useful in research environments as it rapidly evolves to suit each study and its own characteristics. Moreover, this style of leadership provides direction and supervision while encouraging employees to be more self-reliant through participation in decision-making contexts. Importantly, team leaders must be able to delegate to those who can work independently; this practice is not only beneficial for the leader but also for the team, as it favours their development [2]. Regular coaching and honesty are also integral for the growth and independence of the team. On this note, leaders can adopt different styles of leadership according to the readiness of their team members. For example, if a team requires close supervision and constant guidance, the manager or leader may need to make all the key decisions and communicate these to the team. In application to clinical research, this leadership style may be useful when there are repetitive results needed, or the members of the team are at novice level [3]. This can also be challenging to a leadership or management team as research is a fast-paced working environment. If the team is able but unwilling to perform a task, then the leader might adopt a '*selling*' style to motivate staff. In clinical research, this is important in uplifting morale. Whereas if the team is motivated but does not have full ability or perhaps feels insecure, then the leader might take on a 'Participating' style of leadership to guide their team through certain tasks. Lastly, the leader might have a delegating style when the team is able and willing to complete tasks and only requires little guidance. In clinical research, this has been suggested as useful and effective as it is considered a good approach for highly functioning teams. Situational leadership may also provide a framework for members of a research team to develop their skills and improve their performance in a comfortable environment [4]. There are, however, some disadvantages in this form of leadership when conducting clinical research in a hospital environment.

Need theory

Maslow's *hierarchy of Needs theory* is useful in explaining motivation based on the pursuit of different levels of needs at a hierarchical order [5]. This hierarchy starts at the most basic level and moves onto more advanced needs. Historically, it was thought that one level must be fulfilled before moving onto the next, the current school of thought supports that there might be overlap between levels [6]. At the most basic level stand physiological needs where the motivation derives from the instinct to survive. This includes shelter, water, food, warmth, rest, and health. The second level is one's safety needs, in which the motivation comes from achieving law, order, and protection from unpredictable or dangerous situations. At the third level is love and belonging needs, such as those achieved through friendships, intimacy, and family. As social creatures, humans need to receive and give love, and as supported by the need to belong theory this can motivate their behaviour. Conversely, deprivation at this level may lead to mental health conditions [7] such as depression. The fourth level covers self-esteem needs; people can be motivated by the need to gain recognition, respect, and status. This covers both respect from others – such as achieving fame and prestige, and self-respect – including confidence, independence, and competence. The last level, which is self-actualisation needs, is what Maslow [5] claims to be the level that humans aspire to achieve. It covers the motivation for personal growth, which may manifest in obtaining and utilising skills, continued education, knowledge, and talents. Clinical research pertains to this last level as ongoing research allows the discovery of new knowledge following the scientific method. At a societal level, clinical research is able to provide innovative ideas to improve clinical practice, thus achieving self-actualisation through ongoing education.

In an attempt to identify the main sources of competition in a sector, Porter theorised the five competitive forces [8]. This is also applicable to clinical research as different teams within different organisations may aim to publish research findings at the same time. The first of the five forces is competitive rivalry where the number and strength of competitors help determine how profitable an industry is. One example might be the benefits of conducting a research study for a specific disease area within a population. If rivalry in this research area is intense, then a team might decide to attract customer by cutting prices and launching high-impact marketing campaigns. Although this might be difficult, in clinical research, a team may reduce cost in various ways while still protecting efficiency. Second, supplier power is also an important competitive force as it highlights the ease at which suppliers may increase prices. In the context of clinical research, teams may consider the uniqueness of their research aims and the cost of sending the final draft of their research to different publishers. The third competitive force is the buyer's power. This is explained as the ease to switch to a new and cheaper competitor if the number of buyers is low compared with suppliers, in order to reduce cost. Instead, the seller's power increases with more customers and less competition. The fourth force is the threat of substitution, explained as the likelihood of another sector providing the same service in an alternative way. In application to clinical research, it is important to consider other teams with similar a similar research focus and how this can affect publishing. The last of the five competitive forces is the threat of new entry; that is if the new entry's capacity is higher than others in comparison.

Schein [9] has described different levels of culture within organisations and has identified three. The first level is the basic underlying assumptions; these are cultural elements that are difficult to describe to people outside of the team and are better understood by people who have become accustomed to how the organisation works. It might take time for new members of a team to get familiar with them; this is especially true within clinical research, given the different roles of team members and different expertise. Although these assumptions are intangible and not written, team members learn to adapt their work behaviour accordingly, with time. The second level of culture is the esposed values of an organisation, which include the public statements about the values through which they conduct their business. In a clinical research setting, this might involve what is written on job specifications and their website. Lastly, the third level is the artefacts; these are the visible signs of culture within a team. They might include the office layout, how members of a team communicate internally and externally and how they address each other. In a clinical research setting, this follows a hierarchical structure with line managers.

Disruptive innovation theory

The disruptive innovation theory was developed in the mid-1990s by Christensen to explain the challenges and the subsequent changes and novel innovations that may affect an established business system. There are steps through which a new business may move up a market, and this is particularly important in clinical research, within the context of drugs and medical devices. It is important to consider that incumbent businesses develop products to appeal the majority of customers with similar demands, causing them to neglect the needs of the downmarket. This creates an opportunity for a new entrant to address the ignored market and work towards addressing their needs at a reduced cost. Then, if the established business does not respond to the new entrant and continues to provide for the most profitable market, the new entrants may move up the market by starting to offer products for this market, along with the neglected market that they started off with. Therefore, as the new entrant starts attracting the customers of the established business, a disruption occurs, which leads to change.

Bureaucratic theory

The bureaucratic theory is an administrative process that uses a structured approach to perform tasks and procedures within the constraints of rules and regulations. This applies to clinical medicine and reseach as there some are elements of bureaucracy and complexities associated with this sector too [10]. There are seven features associated with bureaucratic theory influenced by Max Weber's approach which is useful for research teams. These can be summarised as below:

- Task division and defined job roles: Tasks could be divided into roles and responsibilities, which allow clear allocation and accountability of tasks to ensure their completion within the designated timelines. The staff allocated to the different tasks should have the relevant experience, skills, and expertise to deliver these. Therefore, the job roles are clearly outlined to maximise efficiency and to develop innovative ideas to optimise research setup, implementation and delivery.
- Hierarchical management: This separates management and administrative duties using a layered approach and could help improve team performance. This type of structure delineates roles and responsibilities, delegation, and communication with clear reporting lines.
- Formal selection rules: This method is useful to develop technical skills and competencies based on education, experience, and training, which are then used to allocate job roles, contractual terms, and salaries.
- Efficiency and unification of process: Employees should be aware of all organisational rules and regulations that promote uniformity an aid the achievement of set goals aligned to the vision. Any changes to the organisational functionality should be communicated and the new processes introduced to the employees.
- Impersonal approaches: This helps maintain objectivity in a workplace, where appropriate. Whilst Webber described this approach as impersonal, this is actually an important component for clinical research team in order to prevent biases and promote evidence-based decisions that can be sustainable and consistent.
- Achievement-based advancement: This approach is highly useful to promote staff retention from an operational perspective. Equally, staff retention also favours good employee relations as career advancement can increase outputs and overall performance in an organisation. This is also an evidence-based and fair way to promote staff.
- Process-driven record-keeping: Governance and regulatory requirements emphasise the need for documentary evidence and processes to demonstrate *'the know-how'* and *'the how-to'* when setting-up and delivering research studies. Meticulous record-keeping is a fundamental component for audits, regular monitoring and inspections for all clinical research studies conducted in the United Kingdom.

Scientific management theory

Frederick Taylor published his *Principles of Scientific Management* in 1911, in which efficiency and productivity improvements were proposed following the scientific method. Taylor suggested:

The remedy for this inefficiency lies in the systematic management, rather than in searching for some unusual or extraordinary man.

Scientific management uses methods to analyse workflows as this theory was initially for factories and mechanical shops. The premise of this theory relies on the development of processes that are scientifically justifiable for each element of a task. To develop the science, objectively gathering preliminary evidence to perform the experiments would be the same premise used to construct processes and/or procedures aligned with the tools required to successfully complete these. Scientifically selecting and training employees to carry out these tasks then becomes a requirement. It is useful to develop skill maps or matrices for each team to ensure that all tasks are assigned to and carried out by the most suitable employees.

There are various advantages and disadvantages of using this method, as shown in Table 10.2.

Behavioural management theory

Behavioural management theory established psychological conformities that lead to increased productivity, such as employee satisfaction, motivation, and feeling valued . A major influence of advancing behaviour is workplace culture and hierarchy. Research

Table 10.2 The advantages and disadvantages of scientific management theory.

Advantages	Disadvantages
Optimal performance with better use of resources	Management controls need planning time
Decreased inaccuracy	Upfront training time required, time delay is a possibility
Decreased autocracy	
Minimised operational disputes	
Time efficiency and better preparedness for regulatory audit and inspection	
Steady improvements can be observed with clear measurables	

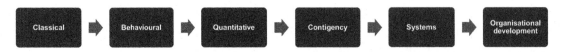

Fig. 10.4 Evolution of management perspectives.

managers that understand the premise to this theory as well evolution of management thought could improve working relationships, staff retention, and overall productivity. Fig. 10.4 indicates the evolution of management perspectives:

The modern behavioural approaches to support workforce commonly use administrative methods led by Human Resources staff. Administrative approaches for clinical research teams could be challenging, hence, the need to take a more pragmatic and evidence-based methods. These can be considered as an adaptive classical approach that underpins behavioural theory, as shown in Fig. 10.5.

10.2 Peer review

The traditional peer review is a process that takes place prior to completing a study and is primarily used to evaluate the concepts and methods associated with the subject of the research. The

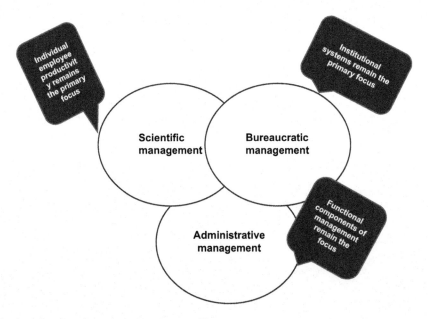

Fig. 10.5 Behavioural approaches used to support workforces.

process began in mid-17th century among academics within Western Europe which was originally referred to as 'the primordial time of peer review'. The Royal Society of London provided peer review on open literature sources and made it available to a range of scholars. The term peer review process was used in the 1960s when manuscripts for publication became synonymous as part of the tenure process in academia within the United States.

The modern peer review process has grown beyond the scope of the biomedical and/or clinical concepts in recent years, as scientific concepts used for healthcare services such as applied sciences and operational sciences, are equally evaluated to ensure the study remains deliverable within the chosen environment. It is vital that the peers review the study from all aspects required to successfully achieve the endpoints. This allows any additional issues to be addressed such as intuitive beliefs of staff associated with the trial conduct, perceptions of the participants, infrastructural problems including but not limited to differences in healthcare systems [11] and geographical locations, and the phenomenon of confirmatory bias which is common in mental health research to be considered. A comprehensive peer review process could aid the ethical evaluation as well as the capacity and capability assessments to further research landscape. To achieve this, a few stages should be completed, as demonstrated in Fig. 10.6.

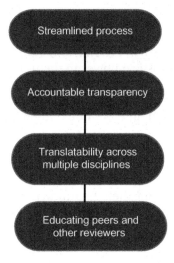

Fig. 10.6 Key stages for a comprehensive peer review.

10.3   Recruitment and retention of participants in clinical research

Currently, there is a worldwide drive to enhance the well-being, health, and wealth through research and implementation. This is present in the United Kingdom, with the National Institute for Health Research (NIHR) sharing their vision of wanting to see 'more patients and health professionals participating in health research' [12].

Clinical research, especially randomised controlled trials, provides the highest quality of evidence for the safety and effectiveness of clinical interventions and treatment [13]. The use of longitudinal studies is imperative for a 'range of applications, including intervention, prevention, developmental, and evaluation studies' [14], making this design one that cannot be underestimated. One element of quality is the recruitment of a required number of participants in order to test the hypotheses with statistical significance. Longitudinal studies require high numbers of participants; thus, the completion of studies depends on the willingness of professionals, patients, and the public to volunteer long-term and/or for the duration of the study [15]. Thus, the more prolonged the trial is, the more of a challenge it is to retain participants.

The challenge of low recruitment rate in clinical research has been highlighted by several studies [16–18]. Evidence suggests that if studies are unable to meet the required level of participants through recruitment and retention, this presents significant implications for the outcome of the study, including adverse consequences on the scientific, economic, and ethical aspects of the studies [19]. The consequences of under-recruitment include a reduction in external and internal validity, with additional impact on statistical power in the trial [20]. Furthermore, if the required sample size is not met, there is an increased chance of type II error occurring, which would lead to conclude there is no difference between interventions when in fact a difference there might be [21].

Prolonged or untimely patient recruitment through the extension of the recruitment phase is a common occurrence. McDonald et al.'s [22] review of 112 clinical trials found that 54% of those had their recruitment period lengthened. However, prolonged recruitment in a trial has economic consequences and could result in an increased direct cost for the trial [23] and/or negatively impacting on the commitment of those already recruited to partake in the trial [24]. This also could raise issues of low enthusiasm and morale within the staff workforce due to uneven caseloads, and, in turn, result in the premature discontinuation of the trial [25]. Additionally, there are ethical consequences to an extended recruitment period as this could cause delays and impact on the administration of effective therapy to the target population, while exposing trial participants to risks [26]. Hence, the ability to successfully recruit participants in a timely manner for clinical research is paramount to the success of research.

Nevertheless, less than half of all clinical trials are able to reach the target recruitment number [27]; this makes recruitment and retention of patients a top priority [27–30]. This topic has been the focus of previous projects, such as for instance one study by Tudur et al. [31], who conducted an online Delphi survey with Clinical Trial Unit Directors on recruitment. They found a consensus of 83% of directors stating recruitment is the highest priority for clinical research, with methods to minimise attrition selected as critical by 71% of responders.

Retention of participants in trials is another challenge that threatens the ability to conduct clinical research [32,33]. It is often referred to as 'attrition', with a broad definition as the failure of participants to continue in the study following enrolment [34]. The attrition rates from several studies have a broad range from 5% to 70% [14]. Attrition is inevitable within clinical research; however, when the rate exceeds 20%, bias is to be expected in the results [35]. This poses serious consequences on the internal and external validity of trials, due to the constant altering in numbers of participants in the experimental and control arm [24]. Moreover, retention could potentially impact on and reduce the overall sample size of the study, thus affecting the statistical power of the trials [36].

10.4 Challenges in recruitment and retention

As mentioned, recruitment of a sufficient number of participants within the allocated time period is a constant obstacle when conducting clinical research. One of the major reported downfalls of the recruitment phase is the phenomenon known as 'Lasagna's Law' [23] or referred to as 'funnel effect of recruitment', whereby researchers and clinicians tend to overestimate the number of patients who meet the set of inclusion criteria and willingness to participate in trials [37]. Evidence by Eder [38] states that a meagre 10% of potential participants pass successfully through the 'recruitment funnel'. The response rate for trials can be significantly low [33], as shown in a review of published GP studies that pointed out the true situation is actually worse due to surveys with a low response rate not likely to be published [39].

10.5 Contextual factors

Contextual factors include culture, funding, political issues, and community practices. For example, a contextual factor that needs to be considered is the lack of involvement of minority groups in clinical research. For example, many clinical trials have fewer South Asian participants than expected, which undermines the government's NHS plan for tackling inequalities and its core principle of providing culturally appropriate and accessible care for different groups and individuals [40]. There are several barriers to an inclusive participation in clinical trials, including: trial burden, treatment preference, and moral views.

For instance, for women from ethnic minority, the importance of modesty can represent a cultural barrier and impact on recruitment for certain clinical trials. American-Indian women place sexual privacy on the highest value, with many individuals showing clear signs of being uncomfortable when undergoing somewhat invasive procedures such as Pap smear tests or breast examinations [41]. This finding was reflected in an investigation on four clinical trial studies that found no racial difference occurred in recruitment to the study, apart from a breast cancer treatment trial [42].

In regard to trial burden, participation within trials is often a demanding process for patients as it can involve additional appointments and procedures on top of their usual care. This can cause inconvenience or additional costs, in regard to travel to and from the clinic or medical centre and time off work, which can be an explanation for low retention in longitudinal studies [43]. Another explanation for low retention is that often participants have a strong preference for or against the intervention arm, such as for instance a reluctance to change their current medication or potentially take a placebo or not take any form of medication [44]. Therefore, clinical investigators need to honour these demands on participants and try to minimise their difficulties to enable an improvement in recruitment and wastage of research.

10.6 Participant factors

Studies have shown that certain demographic characteristics of participants such as gender, age, education, and income provide a good indication of recruitment and retention [32,33,45]. Subjects with limited education and from a low income have lower rates of recruitment and retention in trials [32,33,46]. Some researchers have also considered the psychosocial variables involved with participating in trials, such as the potential negative perceptions of trials and the influence of family members' views on participation [44]. In addition, some trials deal with sensitive issues such as domestic abuse [47], which may have a psychological impact on participants. Furthermore, if the research being conducted is of little interest or not worthwhile for potential participants, it is unlikely that the team will be able to recruit and retain the necessary number of subjects for the clinical trial. This is due to many individuals taking part in research only in order to receive potential additional health benefits; therefore, if the trial is of no interest nor of benefit, recruitment will be low [48]. Finally, practical reasons such as transport and work are cited as challenges to participate or retain in the study, due to the majority of clinical trials being conducted within a week day when many attend work [33].

10.7 Research factors

The research design of clinical trials can have an effect on whether a participant will decide to be recruited and/or will withdraw from the study [24]. Random assignment is a critical aspect of RCTs as the randomisation process distributes errors from extraneous or confounding variables among both the control and intervention arms [49]. It requires participants to be open to assignment to any arm of the trial, such as no-treatment group, intervention group, and standard-treatment group. However, the uncertainties and misconceptions potential participants may have towards the randomisation into the different arms of the trial constitute another barrier to patient participation within clinical trials and can lead to 'fear of randomisation' [50]. In particular, the uncertainty surrounding the randomisation process was shown in a questionnaire study in 299 Finnish breast cancer patients. Almost 51% of the sample thought the doctor involved in the study chose their treatment, whilst 23% were aware they had been randomised and able to explain the method of treatment allocation [51]. It is clear that the confusion and misunderstanding of the randomisation process can lead to the inability for potential participants to comprehend the scientific basis for clinical trials.

10.8   Strategies to improve recruitment and retention

From the above discussion, it is evident that there are a multitude of factors such as cultural, personal, environmental, and research-related elements that contribute to whether an individual will decide to participate in a clinical trial. An overview of the strategies that could improve recruitment and retention is discussed below.

10.9   Participant-related barriers

To improve participants' recruitment and retention, clinical investigators need to identify, implement, and evaluate strategies that aim to diminish barriers that prevent individuals from participating into research studies. This is so investigators can better help and support potential participants by ensuring treatment conditions and data handling are suitable and convenient for them. Intangible incentives include the continuity of an already established participant/research relationship, reminder letters to non-respondents, and the perception of receiving additional care when enrolled in a clinical trial all operate as incentives [52]. Matsui et al. reported that providing patients with an excessive amount of detail on the study reduced the recruitment rates; however, it led to a sustained and more certain rate of participation, leading to a reduction in participant attrition. Additionally, as mentioned, the use of letters alongside follow-up telephone calls has the potential to allow potential participants to feel as though they have the necessary opportunity to consider the proposed research whilst having the chance to have a member of the research team explain the various aspects of the research project. This combination has the potential to result in an increased ratio of eligible participants who agree to partake in the study.

Combining strategies such as for instance the distribution of posters within a clinic setting where potential participants visit while also having a member of the research team present to answer questions, is considered another method to improve recruitment. Through this method, interested patients can make contact with the researcher and have any questions answered without requiring further efforts such as a phone call. The disadvantage of this method is that it is usually not feasible to have research personnel located within such clinics for lengthy periods of time.

Additional strategies to recruit participants include having flexible times for participation andassistance with organising transport to and from the trial site, which is in a convenient location. However, for any of the above strategies to be implemented and show improvements in recruitment and retention, a full assessment of the intended target population, including the environment where the trial will be conducted, needs to occur. The importance of this is shown by Gross et al. [36], who predicted the reimbursement of travel to the clinical trial site by taxis would be deemed as an attractive offer by potential participants. However, due to the limited availability of taxis in the area meant participants could not benefit from this incentive compensation. However, if offered appropriately, incentives can be a meaningful and/or useful method for recruiting participants. Reimbursing participants for either their travel costs or their time involved in participating in research is generally considered acceptable and ethical practice [53].

10.10 Monetary compensation

For consideration are the several deterrents that impact the decision for an individual to participate in clinical research. To combat these barriers, compensation or incentive methods have been used to encourage the initial and continued participation in research, including monetary payments, transport reimbursement, or gifts (REF). Reimbursing participants for their travel costs or their time for being involved within the research is often considered reasonable and of ethical practice (Rudy et al., 1994) [53]. A Cochrane review of incentives to participation and retention in clinical trials found that out of more than 50 interventions evaluated, three trials concluded that the addition of monetary incentives is more effective to increase response to postal questionnaires than no incentive (RR=1.18; 95% CI: 1.09–1.28; $P <.0001$, heterogeneity $P =.21$). Furthermore, the comparison of two web-based trials discovered that the offer of monetary compensation promotes a greater return of electronic questionnaires than no compensation (RR=1.25; 95% CI: 1.14–1.38, $P <.00001$, heterogeneity $P =.14$) [54].

However, there are limits to the parameters of what compensation can be offered, as explained by Gross & Fogg [55], who stated that compensation 'should be sufficiently high so as to encourage participation but not so high as to be coercive'. On this bases, there is a dispute as to the appropriate level of compensation offered to recruit participation. For instance, if the amount of money given to participants exceeds the threshold of a reasonable sum for reimbursement, the provision of incentives for the recruitment and participation in the clinical trial becomes unclear [53]. Gross et al. [36] noted that participants who place monetary compensation as the top reason for participation in clinical research showed reduced retention and higher levels of dropout. Financial incentives may seem enticing and attractive to potential participants; however, the ultimate decision to enrol in a trial is associated with perceived health benefits and relevance to that individual and the community. Therefore, monetary compensation may attract potential participants to enrol within a clinical trial; however, to sustain retention and engagement in the study will be a challenge if there is no perceived benefit or relevance to one's life by continuing to participate in clinical trials.

Therefore, if the questions raised during the clinical trial have been designed by a multidisciplinary team, which includes healthcare professionals and service users, it is expected that the research may spark the participants' interests and needs [56]. By having these discussions, it will enable the concerns raised by prospective participants, to be addressed prior to the start of any clinical trial. Priority setting exercises have gained increasing acceptance as a method in health services' research that involves patients, healthcare professionals, and other key stakeholders. 'Priority Setting Partnerships' aim to identify and give priority to the key research questions in clinical research [57]. Therefore, by addressing the acceptability and importance of certain questions to each of the key stakeholders involved in the partnership, it aims to the overall improvement of recruitment and retention in trials and in turn attaining the conduct of effective research [24].

10.11 Strategies to cultural and contextual barriers

Clinical investigators need to be conscious of the impact that culture may have as a potential barrier to participating in research, with particular sensitivity needed around the customs and values of potential participants. It is imperative for the investigators to have a comprehensive understanding of the needs participants from minority communities may present when considering to participate in a clinical trial. For example, the NHS language line allows researchers access to a service that is able to interpret for most languages. This service was designed to allow researchers to arrange the time and a translator of their choice. Although the language line cannot provide an interpreter to attend the clinical trial in person, it is an under-utilised service that could be a solution to the potential language barrier, and a facility that should be promoted so more researchers are made aware of its existence. Another novel resource is the specialist clinical trial information centre that offers facilities for translation and interpreters for languages 24 hours a day. These centres have the resources to provide packs and information to aid clinical investigators in the optimum ways to recruit individuals from different ethnic minority communities.

Furthermore, a strategy to improve clinical trial participation is direct community recruitment. This strategy involves directly targeting ethnic minority communities through several platforms including, Prime TV, Zee TV, and South Asian radio stations and newspapers that have a large number of readers. As religion holds great importance in many ethnic minority communities, especially in the older generations, direct recruitment by building a relationship and contacts with mosques, gurdwaras, and temples for the promotion of clinical trial participation may also improve recruitment.

10.12   Tackling research-related barriers

When planning a clinical trial, thorough consideration is needed in regard to recruitment and retention. A conceptual framework of recruitment strategies and how to proceed within the study should be included in the planning stage of a clinical trial. To evaluate which strategies are shown to be effective would be beneficial for researchers to aim to conduct a clinical trial [58]. This view was echoed by Treweek et al. [59] in the Cochrane review, whereby they stated that rather than developing and evaluating new strategies, the current evidence of existing strategies should be improved by conducting replicate evaluations.

During the recruitment phase, sufficient time and staff members need to be employed for a successful recruitment, with additional consideration needed for time and staff when recruiting from ethnic minority communities. Targets for the recruitment phase need to be defined and monitored to assess the outcomes of the recruitment period [45]. Moreover, by consolidating contact information of the recruited participants such as their national insurance, will aid in locating those individuals if attrition is high [60].

10.13   Recruitment methods

There has been an increase in the emloyment of a variety of methods to recruit participants for trials [33]. The common strategies used to improve recruitment are news bulletins, letters, and contacting potential participants via the telephone [64]. Combining strategies, such as sending an invitation letter followed-up by a telephone call, may enable potential participations to consider what the clinical trial is researching while being provided with a platform to speak to a member of the clinical staff team to understand the research further. This combination may produce an increase in the number of potential participants agreeing to enrol in the clinical trial. When utilising direct contact as a means to recruit participants, it is advised that this is carried out by clinical staff, after requesting the permission. This allows the potential participant to still gain a rounded understanding of the clinical trial without feeling the pressure to enrol immediately as a participant. The active method of recruitment will yield a representative sample of the target population and improved retention rates when compared with passive methods [24].

The close contact and regular information provided by members within the research team are deemed very important to potential participants. The importance of the first contact with the research team was also commented on by Kauer et al. [60] within their (REF) study of a paediatric trial in an acute setting. The individual that is responsible for the first contact must be comprehensive in the rationale for the clinical trial, the aim and the process of the study, with the ability to answer any concerns raised by the potential participants [24]. Moreover, the effort participants put in trying to understand the multistage trial should be met with encouragement and cooperation from the research team.

10.14 Informed consent

Our study found some of the key principles to reducing waste in future studies and simplifying research-related procedures both for recruitment and follow-up [25]. In particular, the informed consent process must be comprehensive and comprehensible; this is especially important to support the patient (or the next of kin) to make an informed decision. Moreover, the entry criteria should be adjusted and appropriate to the group one intends to study and it should be possible to coordinate these follow-ups with the clinical follow-up. Research must be integrated into the day-to-day work of the clinic [26].

The protocol and informed consent process should be simple and the study-related follow-up should be coordinated with the clinical follow-up. They also highlighted the importance of the availability and encouraging support of the central team in the event of questions.

10.15   Participant information sheet (PIS)

Given the impact of attrition of participants, it is a necessity that retention be considered during the recruitment phase of the trial in order to avoid research wastage by participants who are unable to adhere for the whole duration of the study. Within the Participant Information Leaflet, it is important to reiterate patients' right to withdraw at any time without penalty and without giving a reason. Many teams fail to include key information in the PIS that might reduce unnecessary patient attrition or help assess its impact on the trial.

Furthermore, educating participants about the importance of retention could positively impact both patient withdrawal and loss within follow-up rates and should be implemented alongside other strategies. In the absence of information on the impact of attrition withdrawal can seem inconsequential, increasing the likelihood of patients choosing to withdraw before or instead of voicing concerns or discussing alternatives with clinical staff.

On this basis, it is recommended that staff emphasise the need to talk to the clinical care team at an early stage if problems emerge. For example, the wording can be along the lines of 'if you develop any concerns over participating in the trial please talk to your doctor or nurse to discuss these and the different options available to you'. Informing patients that the team may ask them why they want to stop taking part can be helpful, alongside clearly describing patient withdrawal and making the distinction between premature discontinuation of treatment and stopping all study involvement (complete study withdrawal). Finally, it is important to explain the value of data collection and highlight any options for unobtrusive data collection, e.g. through routine records.

References

[1] Hersey P, Blanchard K. Life cycle theory of leadership. Train Dev J 1969;23:26–35.
[2] Treweek S, Pitkethly M, Cook J, Fraser C, Mitchell E, Sullivan F, et al. Strategies to improve recruitment to randomised trials. Cochrane Database Syst Rev 2018;2, Mr000013.
[3] Chalmers I, Bracken MB, Djulbegovic B, Garattini S, Grant J, Gulmezoglu AM, Ioannidis JPA, Oliver S. How to increase value and reduce waste when research priorities are set. Lancet 2014;383:7–16.
[4] Rabarison K, Ingram RC, Holsinger Jr JW. Application of situational leadership to the national voluntary public health accreditation process. Front Public Health 2013;1:26. https://doi.org/10.3389/fpubh.2013.00026.
[5] Maslow AH. A theory of human motivation. Psychol Rev 1943;50(4):370–96. https://doi.org/10.1037/h0054346.

[6] Hodge FS, Weinmann S, Roubideaux Y. Recruitment of American Indians and Alaska natives into clinical trials. Ann Epidemiol 2000;10:S41–8.

[7] Gregory MA, Legg NK, Senay Z, Barden J-L, Phiri P, Rathod S, et al. Mental health and social connectedness across the adult lifespan in the context of the COVID-19 pandemic. Can J Aging/La Revue canadienne du vieillissement 2021;40(4):554–69. https://doi.org/10.1017/S0714980821000477.

[8] Porter ME. Competitive Strategy. Meas Bus Excell 1997;1:12–7. https://doi.org/10.1108/eb025476.

[9] Schein EH. Coming to a new awareness of organizational culture. Sloan Manage Rev 1984;25(20).

[10] Delanerolle G, Ebrahim R, Goodinson W, Elliot K, Shetty A, Phiri P. The emperors of scientific versatility that influenced clinical medicine. Authorea: Dr Golding Bird and Nikola Tesla; 2021. https://d197for5662m48.cloudfront.net/documents/publicationstatus/60024/preprint_pdf/28f8cc03167a10e4cb30150d78b70474.pdf.

[11] Delanerolle G, Goodison W, Elliot K, Goroszeniuk T, Phiri P, Shetty A. Medical technologies; could this be the "glue" to improve the relationship between health professionals, patients and healthcare systems? A perspective. Psychol Psychology Res Int J 2021;6(1), 000271. https://doi.org/10.23880/pprij-16000271.

[12] Department of Health. Best research for best health – a new national health research strategy. London: Department of Health; 2006.

[13] Haynes R, Bowman L, Rahimi K, Armitage J. How the NHS research governance procedures could be modified to greatly strengthen clinical research. Clin Med 2010;10(2):127–9.

[14] Marcellus L. Are we missing anything? Pursuing research on attrition. Can J Nurs Res 2004;36:82–98.

[15] Patel MX, Doku V, Tennakoon T. Challenges in recruitment of research participants. In: Advances in psychiatric treatment, vol. 9; 2003. p. 229–38.

[16] Lovato LC, Hill K, Hertert S, Hunninghake DB, Probstfield JL. Recruitment for controlled trials: literature summary and annotated bibliography. Control Clin Trials 1997;18:328–57.

[17] Prescott RJ, Counsell CE, Gillespie WJ, Grant AM, Russell IT, Kiauka S, Colthart IR, Ross S, Shepherd SM, Russell D. Factors that limit the quality, number and progress of randomized controlled trials. Health Technol Assess 1999;3:1–143.

[18] Puffer S, Torgerson D. Recruitment difficulties in randomised controlled trials. Control Clin Trials 2003;24:214–5.

[19] Gross D, Fogg L. Clinical trials in the 21st century: the case for participant-centered research. Res Nurs Health 2001;24:530–9.

[20] Bower P, Brueton V, Gamble C, Treweek S, Smith CT, Young B, Williamson P. Interventions to improve recruitment and retention in clinical trials: a survey and workshop to assess current practice and duture priorities. Trials 2014;15:399. https://doi.org/10.1186/1745-6215-15-399.

[21] Kim HY. Statistical notes for clinical researchers: type I and type II errors in statistical decision. Restor Dent Endod 2015;40(3):249–52. Tudur-Smith C, Hickey H, Clarke M, Blazeby J, Williamson P. The trials methodological research agenda: results from a priority setting exercise. Trials 2014;15:32. https://doi.org/10.1186/1745-6215-15-32.

[22] McDonald AM, Knight RC, Campbell MK, Entwistle VA, Grant AM, Cook JA, Elbourne DR, Francis D, Garcia J, Roberts I, Snowdon C. What influences recruitment to randomised controlled trials? A review of trials funded by two UK funding agencies. Trials 2006;7:9. https://doi.org/10.1186/1745-6215-7-9.

[23] Torgerson JS, Arlinger K, Käppi M, Sjöström L. Principles for enhanced recruitment of subjects in a large clinical trial. Control Clin Trials 2001;22:515–25.

[24] Gul RB, Ali PA. Clinical trials: the challenge of recruitment and retention of participants. J Clin Nurs 2009;19(1–2):227–33.

[25] Briel M, Elger B, von Elm E, Satalkar P. Insufficient recruitment and premature discontinuation of clinical trials in Switzerland: qualitative study with trialists and other stakeholders. Swiss Med Wkly 2017;147, w14556. https://doi.org/10.4414/smw.2017.14556.

[26] Watson JM, Torgerson DJ. Increasing recruitment to randomised trials: a review of randomised controlled trials. BMC Med Res Methodol 2006;6:34. https://doi.org/10.1186/1471-2288-6-34.

[27] McDonald AM, Knight RC, Campbell MK, Entwistle VA, Grant AM, Cook JA, Elbourne DR, Francis D, Garcia J, Roberts I, Snowdon C. What influences recruitment to randomised controlled trials? A review of trials funded by two UK funding agencies. Trials 2006;7:9. https://doi.org/10.1186/1745-6215-7-9.

[28] Ioannidis JP, Haidich AB, Pappa M, Pantazis N, Kokori SI, Tektonidou MG, Contopoulos-Ioannidis DG, Lau J. Comparison of evidence of treatment effects in randomized and nonrandomized studies. JAMA 2001;286(7):821–30. https://doi.org/10.1001/jama.286.7.821.

[29] Foy R, Parry J, Duggan A, Delaney B, Wilson S, Lewin-Van Den Broek NT, Lassen A, Vickers L, Myres P. How evidence based are recruitment strategies to randomized controlled trials in primary care? Experience from seven studies. Family Pract 2003;2003(20):83–92.

[30] Sully BG, Julious SA, Nicholl J. A reinvestigation of recruitment to randomised, controlled, multicenter trials: a review of trials funded by two UK funding agencies. Trials 2013;14:166.

[31] Tudur-Smith C, Hickey H, Clarke M, Blazeby J, Williamson P. The trials methodological research agenda: results from a priority setting exercise. Trials 2014;15:32. https://doi.org/10.1186/1745-6215-15-32.

[32] Siddiqui O, Flay BR, Hu FB. Factors affecting attrition in a longitudinal smoking prevention study. Prev Med 1996;25:554–60.

[33] Cooley ME, Sarna L, Brown JK, Williams RD, Chernecky C, Padilla G, Danao LL. Challenges of recruitment and retention in multisite clinical research. Cancer Nurs 2003;26:376–84.

[34] Given B, Keilman L, Collins C, Given C. Strategies to minimizeattrition in longitudinal studies. Nurs Res 1990;39(3):184–6.

[35] Polit DF, Hungler BP. Fundamentals of nursing research. In: Fundamentals of nursing research; 1995. p. 391.

[36] Gross D, Fogg L. Clinical trials in the 21st century: the case for participant-centered research. Res Nurs Health 2001;24:530–9.

[37] Harris EL, Fitzgerald JD, editors. The principles and practices of clinical trials. Edinburgh: E&S Livingstone; 1970.

[38] Ederer F. Practical problems in collaborative clinical trials. Am J Epidemiol 1975;102(2):111–8.

[39] Barclay AN, Wright GJ, Brooke G, Brown MH. CD200 and membrane protein interactions in the control of myeloid cells. Trends Immunol 2002;23:285–90.

[40] Department of Health. Department of Health NHS plan: a plan for investment, a plan for reform. London: HMSO; 2000.

[41] Hodge FS, Weinmann S, Roubideaux Y. Recruitment of American Indians and Alaska natives into clinical trials. Ann Epidemiol 2000;10:S41–8.

[42] Brown DR, Fouad M, Basen-Engquist K, Tortolero-Luna G. Recruitment and retention of minority women in cancer screening, prevention, and treatment trials. Ann Epidemiol 2000;10:S13–21.

[43] Ross S, Grant A, Counsell C, Gillespie W, Russell I, Prescott R. Barriers to participation in randomised controlled trials: a systematic review. J Clin Epidemiol 1999;52:1143–56.

[44] Hussain-Gambles M, Leese B, Atkin K, Brown J, Mason S, Tovey P. Involving South Asian patients in clinical trials. Health Technol Assess 2004;8(42).

[45] Hunninghake DB, Darby CA, Probstfield JL. Recruitment experience in clinical trials: literature summary and annotated bibliography. Control Clin Trials 1987;8(4 Suppl):6S–30S. https://doi.org/10.1016/0197-2456(87)90004-3.

[46] Harris EL, Fitzgerald JD. Eds: The principles and practices of clinical trials. Edinburgh: E&S Livingstone; 1970.

[47] Rosenthal R, DiMatteo MR. Meta analysis: recent developments in quantitative methods for literature reviews. Annu Rev Psychol 2001;52:59–82. https://doi.org/10.1146/annurev.psych.52.1.59.

[48] Newington L, Metcalfe A. Factors influencing recruitment to research: qualitative study of the experiences and perceptions of research teams. BMC Med Res Methodol 2014;14:10. https://doi.org/10.1186/1471-2288-14-10.

[49] Fallowfield LJ, Jenkins V, Brennan C, Sawtell M, Moynihan C, Souhami RL. Attitudes of patients to randomised clinical trials of cancer therapy. Eur J Cancer 1998;34:1554–9.

[50] Hietanen P, Aro AR, Holli K, Absetz P. Information and communication in the context of a clinical trial. Eur J Cancer 2000;36:2096–104.

[51] Aitken L, Gallagher R, Madronio C. Principles of recruitment and retention in clinical trials. Int J Nurs Pract 2003;9(6):338–46.

[52] Royal Institute of Philosophy. Royal Institute of philosophy supplement 87, a centenary celebration: Anscombe, Foot, Midgley, and Murdoch; 2019.

[53] Brueton VC, Tierney JF, Stenning S, Meredith S, Harding S, Nazareth I, Rait G. Strategies to improve retention in randomised trials: a Cochrane systematic review and meta-analysis. BMJ Open 2014;4, e003821. https://doi.org/10.1136/bmjopen-2013-003821.

[54] Gross D, Fogg L. Clinical trials in the 21st century: the case for participant-centered research. Res Nurs Health 2001;24:530–9.

[55] Chalmers I, Bracken MB, Djulbegovic B, Garattini S, Grant J, Gulmezoglu AM, Ioannidis JPA, Oliver S. How to increase value and reduce waste when research priorities are set. Lancet 2014;383:7–16.

[56] Gillies K, Chalmers I, Glasziou P, Elbourne D, Elliott J, Treweek S. Reducing research waste by promoting informed responses to invitations to participate in clinical trials. Trials 2019;20:613. https://doi.org/10.1186/s13063-019-3704-x.

[57] Mapstone J, Elbourne D, Roberts I. Strategies to improve recruitment to research studies. Cochrane Database Syst Rev 2007;2, Mr000013.

[58] Treweek S, Pitkethly M, Cook J, Fraser C, Mitchell E, Sullivan F, et al. Strategies to improve recruitment to randomised trials. Cochrane Database Syst Rev 2018;2, Mr000013.

[59] Bower P, Brueton V, Gamble C, Treweek S, Smith CT, Young B, Williamson P. Interventions to improve recruitment and retention in clinical trials: a survey and workshop to assess current practice and duture priorities. Trials 2014;15:399. https://doi.org/10.1186/1745-6215-15-399.

[60] Kauer J, Malenka R. Synaptic plasticity and addiction. Nat Rev Neurosci 2007;8:844–58. https://doi.org/10.1038/nrn2234.

Further reading

Staniszewska S, Brett J, Mockford C, Barber R. The GRIPP checklist: strengthening the quality of patient and public involvement reporting in research. Int J Technol Assess Health Care 2011;27:391–9. https://doi.org/10.1017/s0266462311000481.
Taylor R. The political prophecy in England. New York Chichester, West Sussex: Columbia University Press; 1911. https://doi.org/10.7312/tayl93968.
INVOLVE Strategy 2012–2015. Putting people first in research. National Institute for Health Research (NIHR), http://www.invo.org.uk/.

11

Research governance and compliance management

Key messages

- The UK Research governance framework is based on the Health and Social Care policy, and subsequent framework.
- The UK has a broad array of regulations, principles, codes of practice, and standards that require adhering to when conducting research.
- Continuous improvement in research quality is a feature of the UK compliance and governance management approaches.
- Transparency and a culture of learning are part of the governance framework.
- A modern set of principles are followed to obtain a single centralised approval system.

11.1 Background

The United Kingdom has a centralised clinical research setup and delivery system where the Health Research Authority (HRA) and the UK Health Departments in England, Scotland, Wales, and Northern Ireland provide a single-approval process for a variety of studies. However, some studies do not fall within the HRA's oversight, and the higher education institutional ethics and governance committees could be used to obtain the necessary approvals to ensure studies are able to continue. Thanks to these aspects along with sponsor oversight, the United Kingdom can ensure a safer way to deliver and conduct clinical research. The ideology of research being overseen by a sponsor and the HRA ensures that research can follow its core functions in order to generate and improve the existing evidence base and reduce risks, and in turn lead to improve clinical care. Policy frameworks and clinical guidelines allow the adoption of a *culture of learning*.

The research landscape has significantly changed due to COVID-19. Moving forward, both COVID-19 and non-COVID-19

Clinical Trials and Tribulations. https://doi.org/10.1016/B978-0-12-821787-0.00007-6

research would continue. Like many other countries, the United Kingdom has a large portfolio of clinical research commitments that will require improved ways of delivery within shorter time-scales where possible to meet the growing healthcare demands. Sustainable, effective, and innovative practices are important to expedite ethical and study setup procedures. A useful method has been the use of digital clinical research pathways where many aspects are remotely conducted to better use capacity and capability. The UK government policy papers for 2021–2022 research implementation plans indicate the efficiency expected from all research conducted in the NHS and academic institutions. The NHS long-term plan, Life Science Sector Deals, and A Healthier Wales and Framework for NHS Scotland indicate the commitment to and expectations from the forefront clinical research.

11.2 Research governance

Research governance plays a role at all levels in clinical research. There are five strategic components that the UK government reports as vital for research delivery, as follows:

1. Streamline, efficient, effective, and innovative research: the importance of ensuring the United Kingdom continues to strengthen and conduct cutting-edge clinical research within shorter timescales
2. Clinical research continues to be embedded in the NHS: yearly growth of hospital involvement when delivering research is a goal for the NIHR. The aim is to develop a pro-research culture among all health and social care staff and for them to feel empowered to support research as part of their routine job roles
3. Patient-centric research: to ensure equal opportunities are provided to all patients in accessing and participating in research
4. Use of data and digital tools: the United Kingdom is increasing data-enabled research and the use of routine data. The use of digital tools and the development of more tools are increasing to meet the demands of a rapidly evolving research landscape
5. Sustainable and supported research workforce: staff retention, progression, equal opportunities and pay scales are an issue with research professionals across the breadth of non-commercial and commercial research

These are realistic goals and serve as a foundation to develop and future proof the UK research landscape in order to produce high-quality research. In addition, in the light of the success stories of COVID-19, the UK Clinical Research Recovery,

Resilience and Growth (RRG) programme has been set to continue to promote flexible approaches to conducting research and improving close collaborations in the research community.

There are different governance tools used in clinical research, as whilst the primary framework within the United Kingdom is unified, institutional practices and policies vary. Variations are observed inter-disciplinary, inter and intra-institutionally, and within hospital versus academic governance procedures; however, this is a reality that is not confined to the United Kingdom alone. This creates time delays in receiving approvals when conducting research.

The UK's ambitious initiatives to grow research require efficient processes to ensure governance is maintained, especially when conducting digital clinical trials or collecting routine clinical data for real-world clinical trials or epidemiology studies. Creating data-enabled outputs with flexible trial delivery models requires the use of adaptable performance measures instead of conventional recruitment targets. Most NHS sites that reach their recruitment targets still lose fundings from the NIHR because of this, thus suggesting that better evaluation methods are required. Some academic sites use hub-and-spoke models and share resources to build capacity, which are not always reflected in funding allocations when recruitment is used as a performance measure. Innovative trial delivery models require novel performance measures that can also improve recruitment numbers when using remote methods.

The use of digital platforms is another aspect that requires attention as at present there are multiple approvals required to obtain clinical data in such a way in epidemiology studies and clinical trials. The quality of the dataset is based upon the manner in which the construct of the data has been discussed in detail in the data science chapter [1].

Whilst there is some recognition of these facets among health policy-makers, current policies require devolved responsibilities since the United Kingdom has identified nations with distinct ownership of research governance and approval procedures. To truly support the UK research ambitions, seamless and linear processes with better recognition for researchers should be made available. For example, providing outreach research clinics could better serve a growing and demanding population with complex healthcare requirements that will influence the type of research being conducted.

11.3 Research compliance management

Research compliance management means different things to different staffing groups working in clinical research. In particular, compliance management is dependent upon the healthcare and academic organisation structure. Typically, adherence to regulations, policies, standards, and legislations is covered within the research management realm.

High-level oversight and management of research compliance are completed by the organisational sponsorship teams.

References

[1] Phiri P, Cavalini H, Shetty S, Delanerolle G. Digital maturity consulting and strategizing to optimise services: an overview. JMIR Preprints 2022;37545.

Further reading

Delanerolle G, Riga E, Thayanandan T, Griffiths J, Lawson J, Roberts S, et al. Women in science: achievements and ambitions. Br J Neurosci Nurs 2021;17(1):13–6. https://doi.org/10.12968/bjnn.2021.17.1.13.

Stanford Encyclopedia of Philosophy. Harriet Taylor Mill. Available from: http://plato.stanford.edu/entries/harriet-mill/.

Sommerville. University of Oxford. Hidden from History: Harriet Taylor and John Stuart-Mill – the love affair that made modern liberalism. Available from: https://www.some.ox.ac.uk/news-events/event/hidden-from-history-harriet-taylor-and-john-stuart-mill-the-love-affair-that-made-modern-liberalism/.

Hall JA, Salgado R, Lively T, Sweep F, Schuh A. A risk-management approach for effective integration of biomarkers in clinical trials: perspectives of an NCI, NCRI, and EORTC working group. Lancet Oncol 2014;15(4):e184–93. https://doi.org/10.1016/S1470-2045(13)70607-7.

12

Audits and inspections

Key messages

- Conducting regular audits and inspections is an important component to ensure scientific rigour, safety, and human rights are maintained
- Institutional audit programmes should be conducted by the sponsor's office to ensure appropriate oversight on conducting studies effectively and efficiently
- Inspections readiness is key to ensuring research staff remain prepared to deliver these as required
- The regulatory and legislative landscape for conducting research in the United Kingdom is key to the successful delivery
- Documentation, following process, and procedures are key to the optimal delivery of audits

12.1   Background

One of the pillars of scientific research is the reliability of results and data generated. With this aim, quality assurance is an essential element of any research, which demonstrates the commitment of management and researchers [1]. In order to deepen our knowledge of quality assurance in research, we must understand what this is first. In a nutshell [2], quality assurance is aimed at ensuring that research data and reports are accurate, complete, and transparent; this allows for the reconstruction and reproduction of data when necessary. In addition, Standard Operating Procedures (SOPs) are an essential source for keeping researchers informed about the defined and agreed methodology that must be followed to ensure consistency across researchers. The following diagram outlines how quality assurance practices work (Fig. 12.1).

The term quality control can be defined as the procedures that the research team puts into the quality and accuracy of the data used as well as the methodologies chosen for a specific [3] study. In the context of quality research, we can define quality control

Clinical Trials and Tribulations. https://doi.org/10.1016/B978-0-12-821787-0.00005-2

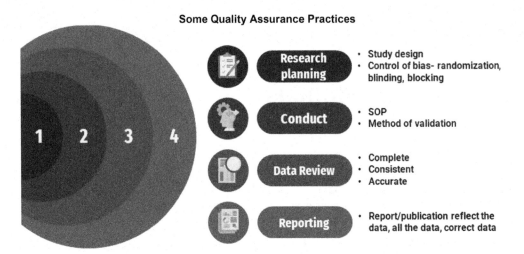

Fig. 12.1 Quality assurance practices.

and quality strategies so that data are maintained, and the research is reliable and secure at all stages of the quality project. There are several reasons for the quality control process to be implemented in research, the most obvious of them being that it ensures the research objective is rigorously reached and the reproducibility of data is possible. Other factors are also important such as [4] Internal Review Committees, funding agencies, and other organisations overseeing and regulating research activity. It is usually arranged that quality assurance and control procedures are implemented in project workflows to ensure that all policies are followed, and disbursed funds are directed to well-organised and planned [5] projects (Fig. 12.2).

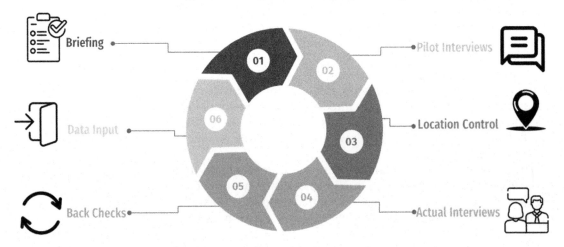

Fig. 12.2 Various quality assurance policies.

Risk assessment

Over 2400 years ago, the Athenians valued their ability to assess risk before making decisions [6]. However, within the scientific field, risk analysis and maintenance are relatively new [7] having a history of about 50 years. Sophisticated risk assessments and developing risk management methods have become part of clinical research over the last decade given the growing number of complex interventions developed to diagnose and treat equally complex conditions. Risk assessments by definition have now become a mandatory component used in clinical trials and considered as good practice to be used in epidemiology and other types of studies. Risk assessments are vital from a quality assurance and governance perspective as they ensure the safety of the studies conducted. The sponsoring organisation and the research teams conducting the studies are held responsible for completing risk assessments and managing any ongoing risks in a study.

Comprehensive risk assessments comprise risk characterisation across all processes and procedures conducted and included in a protocol, in addition to the specific product and cohort associated risks. Regulatory-based monitoring (RBM) systems can assist with developing mitigation plans and also developing RBM tools. RBM tools are based on systematic risk methodology assessments (RMAs) comprising a scientific and clinical basis. RMA theories have been used to develop software such as *R foundation for Statistical Computing* [6–9] to describe risk assessment processes by way of conducting risks analyses and visualisation tools. Scoring algorithms used produce radar plots and provide computed risk scores for the overall trial. RMA tool remains novel with limited use despite this approach reducing bias decision-making when reporting risk categorisation in risk assessment. An example of a risk assessment scoring system is shown in Table 12.1.

The scoring algorithm visuals can be quantified as follows (Fig. 12.3).

Area A$= 0.5 \times$ input (impact) $\times$ input (detectability) $\times \sin (120)$; Area B $= 0.5 \times$ input (impact) $\times$ input (detectability) $\times \sin (120)$; Area C$= 0.5 \times$ input (impact) $\times$ input (detectability) $\times \sin (120)$

Total risk$=$ A1 $+$A2 $+$ A3 $=$ A4

A4 $=$ risk assessment

The risk assessment would also be helpful in developing a trial or study-specific *risk tolerance* threshold that would aid further when adjusting and reporting relative risks, statistically in relation to the interventions. Risk adaptation is encouraged and the

Table 12.1 Example of risk assessment scoring system.

Risk summary	Risk category	Score
Impact	Participant safety	3
	Reliability	2
	Protocol guidelines and adherence	1
Probability	Very likely	5
	Likely	4
	Like probability	3
	Unlikely	2
	Very unlikely	1
Detectability	Site level monitoring	2
	Remote monitoring	1

Risk A

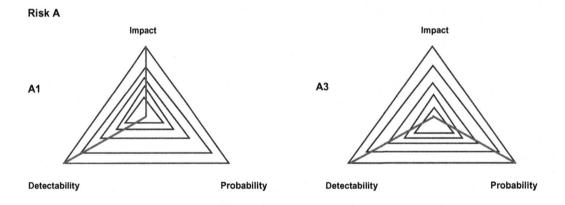

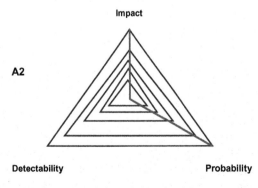

Fig. 12.3 Scoring algorithm visuals for risk assessment.

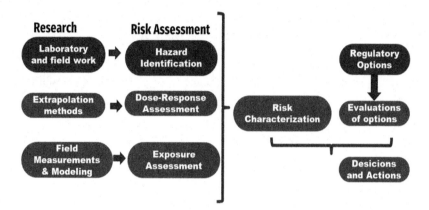

Fig. 12.4 The links between Risk Assessment and Risk Management and the essential role of Research in the overall process. Adapted from NRC/NAS 1983.

MHRA has implemented a scheme based on a risk categorisation approach for drug-based clinical trials. Risk categorisation of a drug is based on the medical purpose and marketing status. In addition, risks associated with the trial design, procedures, and population would also be considered. The MHRA's risk adaptation approach forms the basis to developing processes to manage any ongoing risk that Quality Assurance (QA) staff can identify through ongoing monitoring plans and audits (Fig. 12.4).

12.2   Audits

Audits are performed by sponsors, independent authorities, and regulatory organisations to check and verify that the conduct of clinical research activities is in line with the UK's regulations and sponsor standard operating procedures (SOPs). There are multiple types of audits (Table 12.2) and these are generally based on risk assessments completed and in proportion to complexity of the studies.

Audit compliance in the United Kingdom is commonly conducted in line with the following regulations:

- Medicines for Human Use (Clinical Trials) Regulations 2004, incorporating amendments (2006) from the EU Directive 2005/28/EC on GCP
- Data Protection Act 2018 and General Data Protection Regulation (GDPR, Europe)
- UK policy framework for health and social care research
- Guideline for Good Clinical Practice

Table 12.2 Different types of audits.

Audit type	Description	Scope	Usability
System	Assessing the functionality including manual processes and/or databases and/or quality management systems	Pharmacovigilance, statistical analysis and monitoring, routine healthcare data systems, healthcare data use with epidemiology outcomes and clinical trial monitoring can all be considered within the scope of a system audit. Local standard operating procedures and quality plans would formulate part of the scope of this type of audit. Selection criteria for systems can be complex and therefore the scope may be amended during the audit. Factors that could impact the scope include safety data reporting, consenting procedures used, recommendations about data monitoring and reference safety information change, sponsorship/GCP compliance and process control including changes to quality metrics data as well any findings from monitoring reports that raise questions around process stability	Applicable to clinical trials and epidemiology studies
Facility	Assessing the operational and strategic management of a particular department, clinical trials unit, clinical research facility and research unit	All operational and strategic components such as the daily running of research and their leadership team's ability to manage operations would be reviewed	Applicable to all research studies conducted within the scope of the department, clinical trials unit, clinical research facility and research unit

Table 12.2 Different types of audits—cont'd

Audit type	Description	Scope	Usability
Third-party	Assessing the services provided by a third party	The investigational medicinal product or medical device provider, laboratory providing any analysis, clinical trials unit that is responsible for oversight and delivery of a clinical trial in line with a protocol would be within the scope of this audit type	Applicable to all types of research studies
Study specific	Assessing the activities associated with a named study	The entire study is within the scope of the audit	Applicable to all clinical trials and epidemiology studies
Documentation and/or regulation specific	Assessing specific documents and software packages in line with various research regulations such as clinical trial regulations or medical device regulations or Good Clinical Practice (GCP)	Documents that are within the scope of the regulations and/or principles such as GCP	Applicable to all clinical trials and epidemiology studies
Triggered	Assessing specific concerns or risks raised	The scope of a triggered audit is based on the reported concerns such as a serious breach, major findings, whistle blowing and/or multiple protocol deviations including but not limited to system noncompliance	Applicable to all clinical trials and epidemiology studies
Sampling-frame	Assessing studies using risk-based approaches	The scope of the audit is based on the risks recognised and documented within the study setup and conduct process. Risk tools used to manage the severity of risks will also be reviewed to evaluate the effectiveness of the method to manage the reported risk	Applicable to all clinical trials and epidemiology studies

- Institutional study/system-specific SOPs and Working Instructions (WIs)

  Common audit objectives include the following:
- Review compliance of the study/system with the study protocol, GCP, SOPs, and all applicable legal and regulatory requirements
- Identify corrective and preventative actions required within the study/system
- Assess the knowledge of the team involved with this study/system with regard to the study protocol and local SOPs/WIs

  Key documents that are reviewed in all type of audits include the following:
- Trial master file (TMF) or Study master folder (SMF)
- Participant consent documents including access to source documents and/or systems
- Randomisation system
- Staff associated with the study, as per the roles and responsibilities documents
- Local SOP/WI/Template review

Auditors and/or auditor team

Auditors are independent to a research team and most are placed within a sponsorship office. An auditor should be qualified by training and experience, which should be documented (ICH GCP E6 R2-5.19.2). Auditors are responsible for documenting their audit plan, process, and reports, which are often reviewed during inspections, especially in the context of high-risk clinical trials.

Auditors may choose studies based on a number of criteria including risk assessments that may have been conducted as part of a study setup, including regulatory required. Sponsors often have an audit programme and regular audits are conducted for CTIMPs, medical devices, and healthcare data-based studies. Historically, the number of CTIMP audits versus non-CTIMPs was skewed although this has changed significantly following the use of routinely collected healthcare data to develop various interventions that may fall within the Medical Devices regulations, as stipulated by the MHRA. Risk aversion is an important facet considered by all sponsors; thus, novel scientific methods such as quality by design have been opted to aid in managing more realistic approaches to auditing frequency.

The MHRA has developed and implemented a risk assessment formula based on risk categorisation and severity driven by the purpose and scope of the study as shown in Table 12.3.

- Catastrophic—5
- Major—4

Table 12.3 MHRA risk categorisation.

MHRA risk assessment	Type A/Type B/Type C		
Category/severity	5–4	3–2	1
Definition	Risk has severe potential harm to patients (volunteers) and/or integrity of data	Risk has potential for serious impact if not managed appropriately on patient safety and/or integrity of data	Risk has little or no potential impact on patient safety and/or integrity of data

- Significant—3
- Moderate—2
- Low—1

There are various other risk factors that auditors would consider as part of developing an audit programme. These include:
- Study population and/or cohort selection, including vulnerable patients, new indications, sample size
- Therapeutic area
- Product characterisation, such as specific risks, adverse events, and serious adverse events
- Applicability of regulations, including international versus noninternational
- Importance of study to future marketing submission, in particular CTIMPs
- Level of experience of the clinical research team
- Confidence in service providers
- Number and nature of outsourcing activities, such as the use of third parties (e.g. laboratories) and associated interfaces for responsibility (e.g. clinical trial units, independent statistical support)
- Level of complexity of study and training requirements (e.g. e-system usage or use of medical devices)

Auditing teams do not work alone and their work is scrutinised by senior management teams within regulatory bodies, independent authorities, and sponsorship teams. The auditing procedure should follow these steps:
1. The status and rationalisation of the processes used as part of the audit
2. Use of any previous audit reports

3. Defining the audit criteria including the scope, frequency, and methods, aligned to the study protocol
4. The type of audit being performed, such as triggered or systems, which has defined criteria and scope. This would also involve the use of access to any monitoring report findings
5. Methods will comprise reviewing of study protocol defined procedures and its alignment to any gathered data into a secure database or physical location
6. Use of the relevant audit tools to provide a score when synthesising the findings for the purpose of writing the report

Auditors and their teams are required to complete the planning template and the final report which should include guidelines and/or regulations that may have been followed, any contradictory procedures used, a checklist for reviewing audit finding validators and a feedback questionnaire. For example, audit reports that use GCP could have the following:

- GCP E6 R2—5.19.3 'The observations and findings of the auditor(s) should be documented'.
- GCP E6 R2—5.20.1 'Non-compliance with the protocol, SOPs, GCP, and/or applicable regulatory requirement(s) by an investigator/institution, or by member(s) of the sponsor's staff should lead to prompt action by the sponsor to secure compliance'.

If there are any noncompliance issues that could affect or have the potential to affect the protection of patients or reliability of the results, the sponsor will be advised to perform a root-cause analysis (RCA) and implement corrective and preventative actions (CAPA). One of the practicalities associated with developing audit summaries is to make preliminary recommendations. Common recommendations audits provide include the following:

- A list of compliance gaps with supporting evidence
- Cross-reference findings with regulatory requirements
- A grading of the findings based on the current MHRA criteria, as shown in Table 12.4

Every audit will consist of a follow-up audit. The purpose of a follow-up audit is to ensure that corrective and preventative actions in response to audit findings have been put into practice by the team. The auditor who conducted the initial audit will also complete the follow-up audit, except in cases of mitigating circumstances. The auditor must ensure that all reparative actions requested are in progress or have been completed by the study CI/system owner or delegated individual. The follow-up audit could be completed using two methods:

- Remotely; In situations where it is possible to review the required CAPAs and other required changes without being on site and through documentation sent to the audit team

Table 12.4 MHRA criteria for grading of findings.

Critical

A critical finding is defined by its capacity to directly undermine the integrity of the entire study. This could be a weakness of, or noncompliance with, a control process which, if not resolved, will cause harm to patients or data integrity and/or organisation reputation. This requires the immediate notification and attention of senior management and clear timelines for resolution. A combination of multiple 'major' audit findings may result in a 'critical' systemic audit finding even though each of the findings is not 'critical'.

For example,
- Where evidence exists that the safety, well-being, rights, or confidentiality of study subjects have been (or have had significant potential to be) jeopardised
- Where reason has been found to cast serious doubts upon the accuracy and/or credibility of study data
- Where approval for the study has not been sought from one or more regulatory agency/body or granted from one or more regulatory agency/body (e.g. Ethics committee, MHRA) but the study has commenced regardless. Where procedures not covered/included in the consent form are being performed or where new procedures have been introduced into the study protocol but participants who had consented prior to their introduction have not been asked to re-consent
- Where following study approval, significant amendments have been made to the study protocol or documentation but no new request for approval has been submitted.

Major

A major finding is defined as one that compromises the integrity of a certain component(s) of the study. Weakness of, or noncompliance with, a control process which, if not resolved, has the potential to cause harm to patients or data integrity and/or organisation reputation. It requires the timely notification and further investigation by senior management and clear timelines for resolution. A combination of multiple 'minor' audit findings may result in a 'major' systemic audit finding, even though each of the findings is not 'major'.

For example
- Where there has been failure to comply with the regulatory requirements; e.g. failure to assess and report SAEs and/or SUSARs accurately and to the correct bodies
- Where there has been a significant unjustified departure from GCP; e.g. failure to provide participants with a copy of their consent form or Participant Information Sheet.

Minor and/or other

Minor

Any and/or other findings are defined as those where the integrity of the study is not directly compromised but represent an absence of due diligence on behalf of study staff towards the conduct of the study. Weakness of, or noncompliance with, a control process that currently causes no harm to patients or data integrity and/or organisation reputation that requires resolution

For example
- Where no definite document management/organisation processes are in place at siteWhere there has been failure by study staff to inform the relevant authorities of amendments to start and stop dates or study specific documents

- On-site; In situations where the auditor is required to attend the office/site of the study in order to liaise with the study CI/system owner or delegated individual and review the documentation regarding the required CAPAs and other required changes

12.3 Inspections

Inspections are conducted by various regulatory and independent authorities. In the United Kingdom, the primary enforcement agency for clinical trials is the Medicines and Healthcare Products Regulatory Agency (MHRA) inspectorate. The MHRA inspects clinical trials and other types of studies of investigational medicinal products and medical devices conducted by commercial and noncommercial organisations. A few other organisations that conduct inspections in the United Kingdom include the European Medicine Agency (EMA) followed within the EU, US Food and Drug Administration (FDA), Health Canada, Swiss-medic, HPRA Ireland, AEMPS Spain, ANSM France, PEI Germany, TGA Australia, ANVISA Brazil, HAS Singapore, WJP, Saudi FDA, National Medical Products Administration (NMPA) in China, and the Pharmaceuticals and Medical Device Agency (PMDA) in Japan.

Given the growing number of clinical research studies conducted globally and the difference in legislations to implement novel interventions, the International Coalition of Medicines Regulatory Authorities (ICMRA) [10,11] was established in August 2020. The ICMRA is a working group aimed at developing remote inspections for GCP and GMP due to the pandemic. ICMRA comprises a policy group as well, which presented initial experiences of changes observed within the regulatory oversight of remote working [12]. A reflection was subsequently published in October 2020. The working groups within the ICMRA have since met regularly to work towards global approaches to conducting inspections in research. They make use of the following terms:
- Remote evaluation
- Remote assessment
- Remote inspections
- Desktop inspection
- Distant assessment

The above terms can be used in the context of inspection documents including activity documents, facility records, and other resources that are considered as work performed for research.

Table 12.5 ICMRA inspection vocabulary and definitions.

Term	Definition
Onsite inspection	Inspections conducted when inspectors are physically onsite
Remote inspection/Distant assessment/Evaluation	Inspections, evaluations or any assessments conducted virtually using technology for communicating, sharing and reviewing and accessing systems without the physical presence of an inspector at the site being inspected
Hybrid inspection/assessment	An inspection/assessment performed using a combination of onsite and remote means
Collaborative inspections	Inspections involving two or more regulatory authorities

Additional definitions have also been developed by the ICMRA (Table 12.5).

ICMRA demonstrates the requirement for risk assessments and risk management on a case-by-case basis including the use of high-quality risk management principle and tool when decisions are made in regard to regulatory oversight. The decision-making process is based on local or international restrictions in order to: manage public health emergencies, protect health and safety of the inspectors, access the source documents and electronic systems, redact documents where safeguard privacy and confidentiality are applicable, review inherent risk associated with the site, type, and need for the product, advise on the inspectee's ability to remotely support the inspection, assure historical regulatory compliance, scope and objectives of the inspection as well as complexity of the activities required, to be carried out within the site. It was established that although digital technology has not fully replaced on-site inspections, it could be used as an *option* in the future. This is linked to certain activities being considered as requiring in-person monitoring, such as data verification and data integrity checks.

References

[1] NHS Grampian. Quality assurance including audit and monitoring. Available from: https://www.nhsgresearchanddevelopment.scot.nhs.uk/quality-assurance-including-audit-and-monitoring/.

[2] Bens C, Davies R, Eitzen M. Quality assurance: a tool for improving research quality and supporting quality culture; 2017. https://wcrif.org/images/2017/documents/1.%20Monday%20May%2029,%202017/4.%202A-00/C.%20Bens%

20-%20Quality%20assurance%20-%20A%20tool%20for%20Improving%20Research%20integrity%20and%20supporting%20a%20quality%20structure.pdf.

[3] Lavrakas PJ. Encyclopedia of survey research methods. vols. 1–0. Thousand Oaks, CA: Sage Publications; 2008. https://doi.org/10.4135/9781412963947.

[4] University of Wiscosin-Mdison. Quality assurance in research; 2020. August 17. Available from: https://researchdata.wisc.edu/uncategorized/quality-assurance-in-research/.

[5] Develop a quality assurance and quality control plan, https://old.dataone.org/best-practices/develop-quality-assurance-and-quality-control-plan.

[6] Tudur SC, Stocken DD, Dunn J. The value of source data verification in a cancer clinical trial. PLoS One 2012;7(12):e51623. https://doi.org/10.1371/journal.pone.0051623.

[7] Baigent C, Harrell FE, Buyse M. Ensuring trial validity by data quality assurance and diversification of monitoring methods. Clin Trials 2008;5(1):49–55. https://doi.org/10.1177/1740774507087554.

[8] U.S. Department of Health and Human Services, Food and Drug Administration, Center for Drug Evaluation and Research (CDER), Center for Biologics Evaluation and Research (CBER). E6 (R2) good clinical practice: integrated addendum to ICH E6 (R1)-guidance for industry—guideline for good clinical practice—E6 (R2), 2018. Available from: https://www.fda.gov/files/drugs/published/E6%28R2%29-Good-Clinical-Practice-Integrated-Addendum-to-ICH-E6%28R1%29.pdf.

[9] EMA Guidance. Reflection paper on risk based quality management in clinical trials, 2013. Available from: https://www.ema.europa.eu/en/documents/scientific-guideline/reflection-paper-risk-based-quality-management-clinical-trials_en.pdf.

[10] International Coalition of Medicines Regulatory Authorities (ICMRA). Covid-19 working group: remote GCP and GMP regulatory oversight inspections, 2021. Available from: https://www.icmra.info/drupal/sites/default/files/2021-12/remote_inspections_reflection_paper.pdf.

[11] Department of Health UK Policy Framework for Health and Social Care Research UK Clinical Trials (Medicines for Human Use) Regulations. ICH GCP E6 (R2) Nov. 2016 GCP auditing—principles and practice by RQA NHS R&D forum; 2004.

[12] Distinguishing Different Types of Monitoring and Audit, November 2008 JRO UK regulations compliance form (part 2), version 1.0 NIHR RSS framework https://www.nihr.ac.uk/02-documents/policy-and-standards/Faster-easier-clinicalresearch/Research-SupportService/RSS%20framework%20docs/Annex%204%20RSS%20NIHR%20Framework%20P0 8%20Oversee%20study.pdf.

Further reading

Bernstein PL, Bernstein PL. Against the gods: the remarkable story of risk. vol. 383. New York: John Wiley & Sons; 1996.

Aven T. Risk assessment and risk management: review of recent advances on their foundation. Eur J Oper Res 2016;253(1):1–13. https://doi.org/10.1016/j.ejor.2015.12.023.

13

Patients and public support

Key messages

- Patient and public involvement in clinical research is important to improve relationships between healthcare professionals and the general public
- Improving patient representation in clinical research studies is vital to ensure research remains scientifically robust and relevant to real-world population requirements
- Ensuring research funders understand the views of patients and the public is an important facet
- Patient advocacy should be viewed as a useful stream to consider when designing prospective research studies
- Public involvement in *real-world-data* based epidemiology studies is important to understand prevalence and incidence, as well as long-term healthcare outcomes

13.1 Background

There has been an increase in patient and public involvement (PPI) in research, including the development of protocol design, the results dissemination process, and the successful translation of interventions to clinical practice [1]. PPI in healthcare dates back to the 1970s in the United Kingdom where various patient and public campaigns emerged due to clinical failing within the NHS [2]. Paternalistic healthcare was the initial concept behind PPI that led to focusing on PPI in safety and quality. Since the NIHR was developed for the purpose of conducting clinical research based on the needs of patients and the public, several other facets have been introduced to improve the delivery of successful research programmes. In recent years, the emphasis on the involvement of patients and the public has increased. Including patients and members of the public has incurred since the 1950s using various schemes including discussions around governance. Patients have increasingly emphasised the need to be

Clinical Trials and Tribulations. https://doi.org/10.1016/B978-0-12-821787-0.00009-X

involved in the clinical decision-making processes and in the development of research that is important to better diagnose and treat conditions. Serious failings within clinical practice such as the Bristol Royal Infirmary and Alder Hey scandal furthered the need for changes in healthcare practices.

In addition, funding bodies within the UK mandate the involvement of patient–public involvement (PPI). This led to the establishment of INVOLVE, a division of the NIHR to promote PPI in research, which includes patient advisory groups that provide valuable feedback on studies. Effective contributions made by PPI groups could increase the quality, relevance, and acceptability of research, as well as any subsequent use of PPI in clinical practice.

For people who have taken part in PPI consultations, the impact of public involvement could be challenging due to a number of reasons. These include differing types of research and environments, people involved and diversity in research processes as well as the researcher's reasons for involving patients and the public, including the impact of carefully considering the issues raised as part of the research question.

13.2   Patient–public involvement (PPI)

Conceptually, Patient–public involvement (PPI) has become a facilitating factor in many funding applications, in turn leading to changes amongst clinicians and researchers around traditional views of PPI in research. The NIHR, as well as various other research groups, have developed useful PPI models as a single best approach is not feasible due to the heterogeneity of research studies [3].

Clinical trials in particular could benefit from the Public Involvement Impact Assessment Framework (PiiAF) which is supported by the UK Medical Research Council funding. The PiiAF group includes members of the public, academics, and public involvement facilitators from the NIHR research network. The discussions within this group aim to promote a bi-directional learning approach which lead to the development of guidelines on how to measure meaningful PPI incorporation. In addition, in 2018, the Scottish NIHR Chief Scientist Office, the Northern Ireland Public Health Agency, and Health and Care Research Wales launched a collective initiative to identify National Standards for Public Involvement. The standards were developed using a public consultation of 700 participants and included the following six indicators:

- Inclusive opportunities
- Governance
- Communications
- Support and learning
- Impact
- Working together

In the United Kingdom, there is a presence for a strong commitment to involve paint and public (PPI) in research. This further covered within the Health and Social Care Act, the NHS constitution, and the National Health Service Act 2006 [4]. The Equality Act 2010 prohibits discrimination based on age, disability, gender, marriage, race, religion, and sexual orientation. This legislation theoretically should prevent any barriers to PPI in research. Despite these, increasing criticism from patients continues in relation to diagnosis, healthcare pathways, treatments, and disease management. There is also an uncertainty in terms of the concept of PPI versus a genuine partnership to be inclusive and involving a diverse array of patients and the public [5]. Within patient safety, PPI literature is primarily led by biomedical research, atheoretical, and inequities. Thus, PPI has been exposed criticisms on lack of inclusivity, diversity, and tokensim. These have led to PPI models being re-reviewed especially if the inclusion in a research project is considered narrow, hence leading to PPI specific research being developed to explore better theories, methods, and approaches to develop better PPI models that can take place in research studies.

13.3 Barriers to patient–public involvement

Involving patients, carers, service users, and the general public within the UK's health and social care research has increased over the last decade. Developing patient–public involvement requires a strong partnership between patients, researchers, policymakers, and clinicians [1,2,6]. Theory behind this partnership has serious consequences as it could improve quality of healthcare research within the United Kingdom and internationally. Initiatives and campaigns to better address barriers therefore should be of importance. There are a variety of barriers associated with PPI from personal challenges for some who may live with a physical and/or mental health condition [7], organisational challenges such as the location and timing of meetings, language barriers, and interpersonal relationships between PPI groups and researchers.

These could be addressed by creating better awareness and dissemination of opportunities using multiple platforms. Raising awareness of opportunities and advertising may sound simple, although from a researcher team perspective, this could add to their workload that may prove challenging to manage multiple pathways when patients and the public contact them to be involved. Thus, the notions of a *double-edged-sword* are an issue that perhaps requires addressing with funding bodies as well. Equally, a lack of formal recruitment procedures to PPI groups means that academic researchers in particular may choose their own preferred staff to include in their research studies than actual patients. Similarly, there may be researchers who have opted for a formal recruitment, but patients may find the process of applying too complicated and to further references, especially since they complete this work mostly on a voluntary basis. Thus, the process of developing PPI and inclusivity should be a transparent and linear process to ensure it is not perceived as a daunting prospect to be involved.

Another facet to this was noted by some researchers to be involving PPI groups to review or common a document only [8]. Whilst it could be argued some may have the sufficient knowledge, others may require further training, thus creating a complex landscape. A good way to address this issue would be to create study specific guidelines and terms of reference (TOR) so that the activities and tasks can be clearly defined and all those in a PPI group equally supported. Another way to support PPI groups would be to provide ongoing support upon request coupled with clear roles and responsibilities document to demonstrate the expectations.

The use of lay language is helpful to most people, even experts from cross-disciplines in the context of some studies. It may not always be possible to transform technical language to shorter versions or lay terms. Notion that research proposals or protocols being too lengthy may be another barrier although, it is important to understand that explanations are required for some clinical conditions more than others. PPI groups have raised concerns around the length of documents, proposals, and the use of 'technical jargon' language. It should be encouraged, where possible to maintain simple language within all study documents whilst maintaining scientific integrity.

For patients that continue to live with a health condition or caring responsibilities, taking part in PPI groups could require more support including emotional intelligence amongst academic researchers and clinicians. Often, for patients living with a chronic condition and/or any long-term health issue or being a carer would mean flexible meeting times and place could be helpful, providing options to those who want to take part in meeting.

13.4 The future of patient–public involvement

The movement to include PPI is growing in the United Kingdom, Europe, United States, Canada, and Australia. For the United Kingdom, the NIHR has pioneered the movement for a strong policy approach to PPI by establishing an integrated organisational infrastructure for its growth, as well as the creation of INVOLVE, a nationwide NIHR funded advisory group that builds on the advancements of PPI. The drive from the NIHR on PPI over the last 10 years, with the work of INVOLVE, has resulted in an environment that has been pivotal to allow PPI to flourish all the whilst ensuring organisations' adherence to the UK standards for PPI.

As the movement for PPI carries on, there continues to be barriers in research including public awareness and attitudes. There is an established awareness surrounding public involvement in research; however, the opportunity for the wider population remains limited resulting in reinforced inequalities and missed opportunities to improve the health of undersevered communities. To improve the diversity and inclusion in PPI, various improvements can be implemented such as utilising alternative sources for recruiting participants including community centres and faith centres, as well as providing clearer guidance on what research is available and how to be involved. Simplifying the information and conducting well-crafted communication campaigns that provide clear information on the research projects will lead to overall improvement in awareness and diversity of research involvement.

As PPI is a valued practice in research, this needs to be echoed within the resources and rewards provided to those involved. There need to be capacity and capability to support relationship building between researchers and patients and members of the public involved to obtain a strong working partnership that is essential for every stage of the research project. Additionally, linked to local NHS and Higher Education Institutional policies and administrative practices, there continue to be delays surrounding reimbursement for participants. These are barriers that further hinder inclusivity and a more diverse PPI as they risk limiting the recruitment only to those who can afford the time and money to be involved. Therefore, there needs to be a shift in viewing PPI groups not just as good citizens but as individuals that play a crucial role in research and, in turn, ensure that adaptations such as in the current payment method, take place to make participation in research easier and more efficient for everyone.

The COVID-19 pandemic has presented new methods to incorporate patient and public involvement within research. Digital platforms have been a vital tool during the pandemic to ensure the continuation of involvement work, providing both new opportunities and challenges within research. They have enabled patients and the public to contribute to research regardless of their geographical location, whereas participation would have previously been restricted to a local area. Being able to expand upon the geographical range of people to involve has allowed the demographics of individuals involved in research to broaden, allowing links with public and patients who may not necessarily have had the opportunity to attend in-person meetings before, such as those with physical disabilities. However, the use of technology to increase patient and public involvement has not come without challenges. Patient and public involvement should not solely occur via remote platforms as this is not a sufficient method for everyone who wishes to be involved in research. In the future, both collaborators and researchers will need to tailor the approaches used to reflect the needs of the targeted patients and public; it is suggested that through a blended approach of digital and in-person participation a wider range of individuals would be able to engage with the research.

References

[1] McCarthy M, Dyakova M, Clarke A. Public health research in the UK: a report with a European perspective. J Public Health (Oxf) 2014;36(2):325–35. https://doi.org/10.1093/pubmed/fdt035. Epub 2013 Jul 28 23896860.

[2] Manoukian S, Stewart S, Graves N, Mason H, Robertson C, Kennedy S, Pan J, Kavanagh K, Haahr L, Adil M, Dancer SJ, Cook B, Reilly J. Bed-days and costs associated with the inpatient burden of healthcare-associated infection in the UK. J Hosp Infect 2021;114:43–50. https://doi.org/10.1016/j.jhin.2020.12.027. 34301395.

[3] Staniszewska S, Denegri S, Matthews R, Minogue V. Reviewing progress in public involvement in NIHR research: developing and implementing a new vision for the future. BMJ Open 2018;8(7):e017124. https://doi.org/10.1136/bmjopen-2017-017124. 30061427. PMCID: PMC6067369.

[4] Martin S, Longo F, Lomas J, Claxton K. Causal impact of social care, public health and healthcare expenditure on mortality in England: cross-sectional evidence for 2013/2014. BMJ Open 2021;11(10):e046417. https://doi.org/10.1136/bmjopen-2020-046417. 34654700. PMCID:PMC8559090.

[5] Mathur R, Bhaskaran K, Chaturvedi N, Leon DA, van Staa T, Grundy E, Smeeth L. Completeness and usability of ethnicity data in UK-based primary care and

hospital databases. J Public Health (Oxf) 2014;36(4):684–92. https://doi.org/10.1093/pubmed/fdt116. Epub 2013 Dec 8 24323951. PMCID:PMC4245896.

[6] Paddock K, Woolfall K, Frith L, Watkins M, Gamble C, Welters I, Young B. Strategies to enhance recruitment and consent to intensive care studies: a qualitative study with researchers and patient-public involvement contributors. BMJ Open 2021;11(9):e048193. https://doi.org/10.1136/bmjopen-2020-048193. 34551943. PMCID:PMC8461270.

[7] Delanerolle G, Zeng Y, Shi JQ, Yeng X, Goodison W, Shetty A, Shetty S, Haque N, Elliot K, Ranaweera S, Ramakrishnan R, Raymont V, Rathod S, Phiri P. Mental health impact of the Middle East respiratory syndrome, SARS, and COVID-19: A comparative systematic review and meta-analysis. World J Psychiatry 2022;12(5):739–65. https://doi.org/10.5498/wjp.v12.i5.739. PMID: 35663292; PMCID: PMC9150040.

[8] Heckel M, Meesters S, Schildmann E, Ostgathe C. Patient*innen gestalten Forschung in der Palliativmedizin mit [Patient and public involvement (PPI) in palliative care research]. Z Evid Fortbild Qual Gesundhwes 2020;158–159:107–13. German https://doi.org/10.1016/j.zefq.2020.10.002. Epub 2020 Nov 20 33229253.

14

Dissemination and implementation

Key messages

- Dissemination and Implementation science is a growing applied research field that merges evidence-based medicine and evidence-based healthcare to promote adoption of novel interventions
- Sustainability of novel interventions from clinical research to a clinical practice setting is an important facet to consider at every step of conducting research
- Disease and Implementation models are an important tool to navigate the planning and delivery process of combining and adapting novel research interventions to clinical pathways
- Healthcare professional *buy-in* and *patient acceptance* are key features to consider when developing Dissemination and Implementation models

14.1 Background

Information literacy practice shows the understanding of practices associated with text or social access, information flow, and the role of practice associates with staff. Wenger [1] suggested that practice is associated with relationships, processes, situational awareness, conflict resolution, and addressing artefacts. Therefore, practice could be characterised as an intertwined process-driven element which is underpinned by the know-how, understanding, motivational knowledge, and emotional intelligence. This also leads to improvements in information literacy. Transformation of scientific evidence in pragmatic terms has a number of processes and is collectively known as research translation. Terminology used in this context overlaps with three key definitions as shown in Table 14.1.

Practice theories currently published demonstrate a number of features including that knowledge is relational as such a

Clinical Trials and Tribulations. https://doi.org/10.1016/B978-0-12-821787-0.00002-7

Table 14.1 Definitions of key constructs.

Construct	Definition
Communication	Communication strategies used to inform, influence and change current practices to improve healthcare. The link between research communication and healthcare is vital to policy makers, the general public, patients, clinicians, and researchers
Dissemination	Distribution of study findings to researchers, clinicians, policy-makers, patients, and the general public following peer-review publication in a scientific journal. There are many modes to dissemination of study findings
Implementation	Strategies to accept, integrate, and sustain novel interventions to change clinical practices

phenomenon brought together with practices, discourses, and tools used to deliver the transfer of this knowledge. A key factor to transfer of knowledge is also interactions amongst the workforce within a particular setting that would need to be influenced by practices and cultural paradigms built up over time. The trajectory of historical, political, psychological, and social influences drives practices and any changes as well as their sustainability. The emphasis of process and negotiation between people is situated leading to the production of positive interactions and engagement. Although a unified theory of practice is lacking, common theoretical factors such as the following are important:
- Knowledge use and translation
- Practice approaches through the use of process and standardisation
- Continuous improvement and sustainability
- Psychosocial and other external factors

Leadership/Management structures often face challenges of steering instructions through change which is convoluted in healthcare for a multitude of reasons, including economic conditions, increase in population, and limitations in meeting healthcare demands. These dynamics are often the result of a tumultuous environment needing a suitable workforce that is able to meet the demand. Hence, this collective knowledge led to the inception of *Dissemination Science* which focuses on promoting evidence-based practices (EBPs).

14.2 Dissemination science

Dissemination science is an emerging area based on communication and translation of research evidence into practice, thus considered as a subcategory of applied science. It is a unique area of the sciences where researchers shape the concepts and methodologies as a direct result of research findings in combination with previous research evidence. Since their initial publications, the American Journal of Preventative Medicine, AIDS, and the Journal of Health Communication as well as various graduate modules in taught degree programmes at universities devote publications to discuss dissemination science. Research dissemination is a key facet of demonstrating findings transparently to peers, other researchers, patients, and the general public. Research dissemination is based on key social scientific principles and closely linked to implementation science. Variations to this concept exist due to differences in research explored and public policy. With the aim of increasing visibility of results, public engagement in science, innovation, and societal trust in research [2], and effective dissemination and communication are vital to ensure positive social impact.

With the recent advancements of technology, we have a series of modern tools to help us share data and results. Social media, for example, has proven to be an excellent and comprehensive sharing tool, through which we are able to target, identify, and connect with influencers who, in turn, can defend the new findings. In addition, websites, blogs, forums, electronic newspapers, and conferences [3] are also dissemination channels that can expand the sharing of research-related content.

Sharing the benefits found in research with other researchers, professionals, and the community at large brings with it a number of advantages; for example, increased awareness and understanding or change in practice [3]. However, for this sharing to generate a comprehensive and significant impact, research results must be made available or shared with people who can use them to maximise the benefits of the research [3,4]. Policy-maker perception is an important part of dissemination as building on existing knowledge is key to further healthcare policies that may impact healthcare practices.

Diffusion paradigm

Diffusion is a process by way of demonstrating novel interventions. Studies that explore this paradigm show a sigmoid pattern, also referred to an S-shaped curve that is mathematically sound [5]. The curve would demonstrate the adoption of the innovation over a period of time. Logically associated propositions undoubtedly would impact these pathways, including the sustainability. There are studies that have demonstrated the S-curve to be cumulative as this could be due to engagement of opinions provided by leaders. More complex statistical predictive models are now used as a way to better understand the potential applicability of an intervention to a healthcare system. Whilst this does not negate the importance of having healthcare staff, including clinicians, on board with using a novel intervention, this data can be useful to disseminate so that a transparent discussion could take place.

Diffusion of innovation theory

Diffusion theory of innovation has evolved over the years and focuses on seven concepts of intervention, namely clusters, societal sectors, intervention adaptation, attributes, reinforcement of contextual factors, leadership opinions, and research studies that are based on implementation science concepts to promote EBPs. In its early years, this theory was defined as follows:

Diffusion really includes three fairly distinct processes: Presentation of the new culture element or elements to the society, acceptance by the society, and the integration of the accepted element or elements into the pre-existing culture.

Ralph Linton (1936)

I once asked a worker at a crematorium, who had a curiously contented look on his face, what he found so satisfying about his work. He replied that what fascinated him was the way in which so much went in and so little came out.

A.L. Cochrane (1972)

Diffusion is a natural social phenomenon that happens with or without any particular theory to explain it. In fact, whether the innovation involves a new idea, new pattern of behaviour, or a new technology, it is also a natural physical phenomenon as well, one that describes the spread of an object in space and time.

D. Lawrence Kincaid (2004)

Diffusion theory does not lead to the conclusion that one must wait for the diffusion of a new product or practice to reach the poorest people .... In fact, one can accelerate the rate of adoption in any segment of the population through more intensive and more appropriate communication and outreach.

Lawrence W. Green, Nell H. Gottlieb, and Guy S. Parcel (1991)

The key composites of the theory are as follows:

- Innovation: details of the innovation are important as the perceptions of the adopter would be driven by the effectiveness, efficiency, and overall operational attributes such as compatibility to the existing operating systems.
- Adopter: ability to understand the innovation and its scalability is an important facet to understand.
- Social system: structure of the healthcare systems is important as this would demonstrate the workplace culture and the sociological aspects amongst the populations that access these organisations. Opinions of leaders and patients are key features of this dimension.
- Adoption process: this is a stage-ordered framework and/or model used to bring awareness, influence, implementation, sustainability, and decision around introducing a new innovation.
- Diffusion system: this is often referred to as *change agents* and can often include behaviour change.

Diffusion methods should also focus on *degrees of readiness* to legitimise the effectiveness of the intervention. The promise of improved efficiency can be alluring to many adopters. Providing cost evaluation reports along with any scientific and clinical information could also be useful to be included in a diffusion method to demonstrate any potential cost effectiveness [6] (Fig. 14.1).

Dissemination models

There are multiple principles that can be used to develop models of dissemination. Firstly, stakeholder engagement should be considered to understand the primary audience and ensure the language and format of the information intended for dissemination could be directed. Secondly, the potential format that would be favoured by the intended audience should be carefully considered. For example, if the audience involves more patients, using lay language to show the study outputs would be more effective. Thirdly, by using the opportunity to disseminate findings, potential networks to exchange knowledge, raise awareness consider focus groups to develop further research and potential inclusion of new researchers to develop working groups. Finally, the context of the research and the influence of the findings by way of those that could act as *champions* of the clinical area impacted from the work would be useful to have discussions medium to long-term following the completion of the study.

There are a variety of theoretical frameworks that indicate strategies for improved dissemination of research to the public

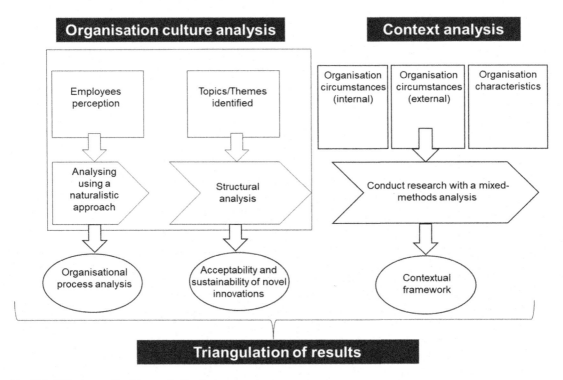

Fig. 14.1 Diffusion method for cost-effectiveness.

and policy-makers. Multiple theories can be used to develop these frameworks that are also referred to as *models of dissemination*. The mathematical theory of communication, matrix of persuasive communication, social marketing theory, and diffusion of innovations theory were used to develop the Model for Dissemination of Research (MDR) [7–9]. The MDR is used to show gaps between targeted readers and the research being disseminated by different features [10]. The diffusion of innovations theory shows the expansion and adoption of new interventions by way of *ordered process*, also referred to as the 'S-curve'. The S-curve approach features dimensions of the message and audience that would demonstrate potential acceptability and suitability of the novel interventions. This furthered by way of the social marketing theory that strategises using four points of price, produce, place, and promotion. This is based upon the understanding that communication alone will not amend behaviours of those that would need to accept the new product [11].

The use of *Broadcast models of diffusion* and *Contagion model of diffusion* is another method that could introduce novel ideas into the healthcare system; social constructs such as friendship, collegiality, structural equivalences. We distinguish amongst diffusion (passive dissemination), dissemination (active and planned efforts to persuade target groups to adopt an innovation), implementation (active and planned efforts to integrate an innovation within an organisation), and sustainability (making an innovation routine until reach obsolescence).

The most common and accepted theories of innovation diffusion [12] assume that people make rational choices about adopting new ideas based on their expectations or life experience, with the exception that some people are inherently open to new ideas. Within this context, anthropologically, *Memetic* and *Mimetic* theory would be useful to support the development of culture. The memetic or meme theory explains the advancement of culture through imitation of behaviours, ideas, and styles which acts as an analogue to biological genes. Richard Dawkins [13], an evolutionary biologist, demonstrated the idea of cultural transmission where the meme is said to propagate itself in a *meme-pool* between individual's brains via the process of imitation. However, Knobel and colleagues [14] indicate that the transmission of information patterns is a direct action of the mentalities of a social group. In other words, genes would play a potential indirect role in the processing of the information. Increasingly, this concept appears to be more in use with the advent of social media to propagate and circulate communications. This has a dimension in the production and transfer of culture. Knobel and colleagues explained key phrases, process or clothing fashion could be included as example of memes. This concept can be extended to research dissemination. Most scientific journals and research studies are publicly available within social media. As a result, readability and viewing the material could be observed to measure public interest. *Mimetic theory* on the other hand is a concept developed by Rene Girard, an anthropologist, to express human desire that would be collective rather than individual, with a four-stage process of *mimetic desire, conflict, scapegoating,* and the *cover-up. Mimetic desire* is a social component and does not include an individual's basic needs such as food and shelter. This leads to *conflict* where people compete for *mimetic desires* leading to *mimetic rivalry.* The *scapegoating* is a mechanism where a problem or an individual is held accountable once the mimetic contagion has spread. Once the problem or the individual has been identified, this would be expelled from the process. The *cover-up* step is the mechanism that moves into a new phase with *change.* It is evident that mimetic and memetic theories are both embedded within the concepts of dissemination of research.

Current literature in memetics suggest patterns of cultural change could be explained without making rationalising decisions as imitation as a basic means of transmitting cultural characteristic could be used.

Oftentimes, sharing through these channels is ineffective, which results in an impact well below researchers' expectations. Greenhalgh et al. [15] developed a robust and transferable model of how to facilitate and disseminate the use of health-related evidence, including how to plan and direct research to the right audience.

Based on Kuhn's scientific paradigms [16], metanarrative review was developed to classify and interpret sources identified in exploratory searches. As the initial unit of analysis, the unfolding of the storyline of a research tradition over time was used. The method itself involves some phases to be considered, as shown in Table 14.2 [16].

Table 14.2 The five phases of a metanarrative review.

1. Planning phase	Assemble multidisciplinary research team whose background encompasses the relevant research traditions
	Present an initial research question in a wide and open format
	Agree outputs with funder or client
	Set a series of regular face-to-face review meetings including planned input from external peers drawn from the intended audience for the review
2. Search phase	Initial search led by intuition, informal networking and browsing
	Search for seminal conceptual papers in each research tradition by tracking the references
	Search for empirical papers by electronic searching key databases
3. Mapping	The key elements of the research paradigm (conceptual, theoretical, Methodological, and instrumental)
	The key actors and events in the unfolding of the tradition (including main findings and how they came to be discovered)
4. Appraisal phase	Evaluate each primary study for its validity and relevance to the review question
	Extract and collate the key results, grouping comparable studies together
5. Synthesis phase	Identify all the key dimensions of the problem that has been researched
	Taking each dimension in turn, give a narrative account of the contribution (If any) made to it by each separate research tradition

Risk communication methods when disseminating new research

Both the 2009 H1N1 pandemic and the 2020 novel coronavirus pandemic significantly and comprehensively altered the population's perception of risk. Some relevant and controversial issues have been raised, such as global health management, vaccination campaigns, and alleged conflicts of interest between government agencies and pharmaceutical companies. The media, as a comprehensive source of impact, often negatively impacts the population from the perspective of risk perception [17]. A survey carried out in Sweden showed that daily listening to the radio from health services and reading the morning newspaper were not associated with fear, whilst daily reading of tabloids and television made people more afraid of the H1N1 virus [17]. Also, in Sweden, another study showed that individuals who are used to reading tabloids and forums and watching television believe less in specialised information sources [18]. Risk perception is totally linked to how much people hear about the disease and the source of information, which usually tends to favour and create panic in the population.

14.3 Implementation science

When poorly planned and consequently poorly implemented, evidence-based interventions and practices tend not to produce significant health effects. In many cases, even when effectively implemented, they still may not offer the expected health benefits [19]. Albeit relatively new, implementation science has many published definitions. Some definitions emphasise closing the knowledge gap, whilst others emphasise the production of generalisable knowledge or locally appropriate solutions [5–11,16,19–29].

Glasgow et al. defined implementation science as the application and integration of research evidence into practice and policy [30]. Further, Allotey and colleagues in 2008 defined it as applied research that aims to develop the critical evidence base that informs effective, sustained, and integrated adoption of interventions by health systems and communities [31]. Later, Peters et al. classified it as scientific inquiry into implementation issues—the act of realising an intention, which in health research can be policy, programmes, or individual practices (collectively called interventions) [20].

Implementation science seeks to improve population health by leveraging interdisciplinary methods to promote the uptake and dissemination of effective, underused interventions in the real world [32]. In addition, implementation science brings evidence-based science to the people who need it, with greater speed, fidelity, efficiency, quality, and relevant coverage.

Curran and colleagues defined an implementation intervention as a method to improve the adoption of a clinical intervention, such as the use of job aids, provider education, and/or audit procedures [20]. In 2008, Sabatier emphasised that some factors can influence the implementation of research, such as clarity in objectives, causal theory, and support for interest groups [21]. Although poorly understood, research implementation is constantly evolving and has contributed to making clinical and public health policies and programmes more effective [25]. We can exemplify as main advantages the positive impact on people's health, contributing to the construction of stronger and more responsive health systems within the realities of specific contexts, improving health management and service delivery, and finally, supporting and enabling communities [27,28].

Implementation research is based on real-world conditions, for example on the facilitators of implementing evidence-based interventions in public and private health systems, as well as on the challenges to their implementation, as well as promoting the use and sustainability of these interventions on a large scale [33]. It does not try to control them [20]. This means working with populations that will be affected by a particular intervention, rather than selecting samples that will not be affected. As an example, we can mention the inclusion of only healthy individuals in a randomised clinical trial.

Implementation paradigms

McNulty et al. listed three methodological paradigms that help in research implementation. These are: (1) use of existing data, that is, make efficient use of existing data by applying epidemiological and simulation models; (2) inclusion of populations with health inequalities in new implementation research, designing new implementation research studies that include, but not only focus on, populations with economic and health disparities; (3) implementation surveys that focus on vulnerable populations, conducting implementation surveys that bring evidence-based interventions to populations that have experienced high levels of disparities [27].

Paradigm 1

Using existing data

The first paradigm is the most simple. It aims to efficiently use existing data, adjusting it through epidemiological modelling and simulation, in order to understand what drives discrepancies and how they can be overcome, based on existing records, administrative and/or formal research studies. The extent of population-level disparities, the mechanisms that can explain them, and the likely impacts of specific implementation strategies on reducing disparities elucidate this analytical approach [27]. To quantify this discrepancy, regression analysis can be used, identifying the prevalence or incidence of a population disorder [5–11,16,19,20,27–34].

Paradigm 2

New implementation research with populations affected by health inequalities

The second method, a little more comprehensive, involves implementing new studies and research methods, without being restricted to populations that present health disparities, such as multilingual communities, racial/ethnic minority, and low-income communities. According to the NIHR, the proportion of racial and ethnic minorities enrolled in home clinical trial research studies is substantially lower than in the general population [35]. Therefore, given the low numbers of these minorities in the surveys, implementation inferences based on an underrepresented population are less accurate than those belonging to the majority population [27]. Unlike clinical trials that target individual-level change and may recruit a defined population, the reality of trial implementation strategies is that they are likely to be administered to a more heterogeneous population.

Paradigm 3

Implementation research dedicated to populations that experienced inequalities

The third and final paradigm is fully dedicated to bringing evidence-based interventions to populations in situations of vulnerability and/or who have experienced high levels of disparities across sectors. When the context to be studied involves low-income populations, low access to education, and all other disparities, there is no other study that can measure how this population is affected [5–11,16,19,20,27–36].

Bringing evidence-based interventions (EBIs) to populations that have suffered or still suffer from health disparities will always be a challenge, especially when they are underrepresented. However, some methods to expand EBI delivery have been developed to allow adaptations to new populations, new health systems, or both [36–38], such as scaling-out. Using existing theories of external validity and multilevel mediation modelling, a logical framework is provided to determine what new empirical evidence is needed for a new intervention to maintain its evidence-based pattern in the new context being studied [36].

Successful implementation is an inherent part of quality research. However, it can be confusing at first, as different variables can affect the implementation process, thus impacting the results and bringing difficulties in discerning the real cause of a result, if adequate measures are not considered from the beginning.

References

[1] Wenger E. Communities of practice: learning as a social system. Syst Think 1998;9(5):2–3.
[2] Marín-González E, Malmusi D, Camprubí L, Borrell C. The role of dissemination as a fundamental part of a research project. Int J Health Serv 2017;47(2):258–76. https://doi.org/10.1177/0020731416676227. Epub 2016 Oct 31 27799595.
[3] How to disseminate your research what does NIHR mean by dissemination? https://www.nihr.ac.uk/documents/how-to-disseminate-your-research/19951#What_does_NIHR_mean_by_dissemination. [Accessed 25 June 2022].
[4] Edwards DJ. Dissemination of research results: on the path to practice change. Can J Hosp Pharm 2015;68(6):465–9. https://doi.org/10.4212/cjhp.v68i6.1503. 26715783. PMCID: PMC4690672.
[5] Green LW, Gottlieb NH, Parcel GS. Diffusion theory extended and applied. In: Ward WB, Lewis FM, editors. Advances in health education and promotion. London: Jessica Kingsley; 1991.
[6] Dearing JW, Maibach EW, Buller DB. A convergent diffusion and social marketing approach for disseminating proven approaches to physical activity promotion. Am J Prev Med 2006;31(4):11–23. https://doi.org/10.1016/j.amepre.2006.06.018.
[7] Shannon CE. A mathematical theory of communication. Bell Syst Tech J 1948;27:379–423.
[8] Weaver W, Shannon CE. The mathematical theory of communication. Champaign: University of Illinois Press; 1963.
[9] McGuire W. The nature of attitudes and attitude change. vol. 3. Reading: Addison-Wesley Pub. Co; 1969.
[10] Brownson RC, Eyler AA, Harris JK, Moore JB, Tabak RG. Getting the word out: new approaches for disseminating public health science. J Public Health Manag Pract 2018;24:102–11.
[11] Rogers EM. Diffusion of innovations. 5th ed. Simon and Schuster; 2003.
[12] Rogers EM. Diffusion of innovations. New York: The Free Press; 1995.

[13] Dawkins R. The selfish gene. Oxford: Oxford University Press; 1976.

[14] Knobel M, Lankshear C. Online memes, affinities, and cultural production. In: Knobel M, Lankshear C, editors. A new literacies sampler, vol. 29. Peter Lang; 2007. p. 199–227.

[15] Greenhalgh T, Robert G, Macfarlane F, et al. Diffusion of innovations in service organizations: systematic review and recommendations. Milbank Q 2004;82 (4):581–629. 15595944.

[16] Kuhn TS. The structure of scientific revolutions. Chicago: University of Chicago Press; 1962.

[17] Barrelet C, Bourrier M, Burton Jeangros C, et al. Unresolved issues in risk communication research: the case of the H1N1 pandemic (2009–2011). Influenza Other Respir Viruses 2013;7:114–9.

[18] Ghersetti M, Odén TA. Top marks: how the media got Swedes to vaccinate against swine flu. Observatorio (OBS*) J 2011;5:135–60.

[19] What is implementation science? University of Washington. https://impsciuw.org/implementation-science/learn/implementation-science-overview/ [Accessed 7 July 2022].

[20] Peters DH, Adam T, Alonge O, Agyepong IA, Tran N. Republished research: implementation research: what it is and how to do it. Br J Sports Med 2014;48(8):731–6. https://doi.org/10.1136/bmj.f6753. 24659611.

[21] Pomeroy C, Sanfilippo F. How research can and should inform public policy. In: Wartman SA, editor. The transformation of academic health centers. Academic Press; 2015. p. 179–91 [chapter 18].

[22] Ciliska D, Robinson P, Armor T, Ellis P, Brouwers M, Gauld M, et al. Diffusion and dissemination of evidence-based dietary strategies for cancer prevention. Nutr J 2005;4(1):13.

[23] Remme JHF, Adam T, Becerra-Posada F, D'Arcangues C, Devlin M, Gardner C, et al. Define research to improve health systems. PLoS Med 2010;7:e1001000.

[24] McKibbon KA, Lokker C, Mathew D. Implementation research., 2012, http://whatiskt.wikispaces.com/Implementation+Research.

[25] Curran GM, Bauer M, Mittman B, Pyne JM, Stetler C. Effectiveness implementation hybrid designs: combining elements of clinical effectiveness and implementation research to enhance public health impact. Med Care 2012;50:217–26.

[26] Sabatier P. Abordagens de cima para baixo e de baixo para cima para a pesquisa de implementação: uma análise crítica e uma síntese sugerida. J Public Policy 1986;6(1):21–48. https://doi.org/10.1017/S0143814X0000384.

[27] McNulty M, Smith JD, Villamar J, Burnett-Zeigler I, Vermeer W, Benbow N, Gallo C, Wilensky U, Hjorth A, Mustanski B, Schneider J, Brown CH. Implementation research methodologies for achieving scientific equity and health equity. Ethn Dis 2019;29(Suppl. 1):83–92. https://doi.org/10.18865/ed.29. S1.83. PMID: 30906154; PMCID: PMC6428169.

[28] Theobald S, Brandes N, Gyapong M, El-Saharty S, Proctor E, Diaz T, Wanji S, Elloker S, Raven J, Elsey H, Bharal S, Pelletier D, Peters DH. Implementation research: new imperatives and opportunities in global health. Lancet 2018;392 (10160):2214–28. https://doi.org/10.1016/S0140-6736(18)32205-0. Epub 2018 Oct 9 30314860.

[29] Greenhalgh T, Robert G, Macfarlane F, Bate P, Kyriakidou O, Peacock R. Storylines of research in diffusion of innovation: a meta-narrative approach to systematic review. Soc Sci Med 2005;61(2):417–30. https://doi.org/10.1016/j.socscimed.2004.12.001. Epub 2005 Jan 26 15893056.

[30] Glasgow RE, Eckstein ET, ElZarrad MK. Implementation science perspectives and opportunities for HIV/AIDS research. J Acquir Immune Defic Syndr 2013;63:S26–31. https://doi.org/10.1097/QAI.0b013e3182920286.

[31] Allotey P, Reidpath DD, Ghalib H, et al. Efficacious, effective, and embedded interventions: implementation research in infectious disease control. BMC Public Health 2008;8:343. https://doi.org/10.1186/1471-2458-8-343.

[32] Eccles MP, Mittman BS. Welcome to implementation science. Implement Sci 2006;1:1.

[33] Sáenz V, Patino CM, Ferreira JC. Implementation research and its role in public health and health policies. J Bras Pneumol 2021;47(5):e20210443.

[34] Ibons RD. Design and analysis of longitudinal studies. Ann Psychiatrist 2008;38(12):758–61. https://doi.org/10.3928/00485713-20081201-03.

[35] National Institutes of Health Monitoring Adherence to the NIH Policy on the Inclusion of Women and Minorities as Subjects in Clinical Research. Comprehensive report: tracking of human subjects research as reported in fiscal year 2011 and fiscal year 2012, 2013. Last accessed January 3, 2019, from https://orwh.od.nih.gov/resources/pdf/Inclusion-ComprehensiveReport-FY-2011-2012.pdf. [Accessed 10 July 2022].

[36] Aarons GA, Sklar M, Mustanski B, Benbow N, Brown CH. "Scaling-out" evidence-based interventions to new populations or new health care delivery systems. Implement Sci 2017;12(1):111. https://doi.org/10.1186/s13012-017-0640-6.

[37] Oliver K, Innvar S, Lorenc T, Woodman J, Thomas J. A systematic review of barriers to and facilitators of the use of evidence by policymakers. BMC Health Serv Res 2014;14:2.

[38] Innvær S, Vist G, Trommald M, Oxman A. Health policy-makers' perceptions of their use of evidence: a systematic review. J Health Serv Res Policy 2002;7:239–44.

15

The future of clinical research

Key messages

- The future of clinical research is dependent upon many facets: key factors such as population and disease demand, healthcare costs, research funding, healthcare system infrastructure, and availability of resources in healthcare organizations as well as higher education institutions
- Understanding, evaluating, and implementing the research landscape from a globalization and locational perspective
- Understanding and informing the changing regulatory and legislative landscape of the United Kingdom to promote better integration of global clinical research
- Improving epidemiology research relevant to the UK population
- Improving diversity and inclusivity in clinical trials that are relevant to the UK population

15.1 Background

Clinical research will continue to evolve at a rapid pace and influence change to optimise clinical practice and healthcare services offered to patients. COVID-19 has further influenced changes in the clinical research arena. As such, further changes should be anticipated.

There are eight themes that would be the primary focus within the clinical research domain, as described below:

- Conduct more patient-centric research
- Increase population science-based studies
- Develop novel methods to conduct efficient and effective clinical research studies
- Improved use of research evidence to improve clinical practice
- Increase use of routinely gathered clinical data to better understand clinical gaps prior to developing research studies and to inform clinical trials
- Better use of digital technologies

Clinical Trials and Tribulations. https://doi.org/10.1016/B978-0-12-821787-0.00015-5

- Sustainable growth and management of conducting research within hospital environments
- Sustainable development of the research workforce with alignment of skills across those working in hospitals, academia, and industry

15.2 Use of existing evidence

Navigating the current research evidence landscape is an important facet to consider in order to build patient-centric healthcare systems that could deliver optimal clinical care. Whilst there are multiple types of evidence that could be used in research, ensuring the accurate use of methods and methodology to report any findings would be equally important. This could assist with combining clinical data with life-course approaches.

Utilising data gathered under research constraints as well as *real-world* data, including those obtained from wearable technologies, would be a holistic view of capturing the *exposome* that could enhance our understanding of clinical conditions as it provides a more accurate view of the patient. This is particularly useful for improving chronic condition diagnosis, management, and treatment. Academia and Industry could also use this approach to gather a richer understanding of the efficacy and effectiveness of current treatments as well as any discrepancies in terms of treatment response over a life course.

There is a conspicuous influence of funding from industry in academia and a consequent 'approach-avoidance' conflict. Academia provides the expertise to carry out research and the patients to be studied, whereas the industry provides the funding. The connection between academia and industry has increased for obvious reasons. The realisation of the commercial value of academic biomedical research, coupled with its rapid and efficient use by industry, is the main driving force here.

15.3 Effectively addressing barriers

Interviews with clinical staff indicated an inadequacy of payments to cover the additional treatment costs associated with research, especially in the United Kingdom. Without such payments met, staff stated there was little, if any, incentive for nonresearch staff to work towards recruiting and retaining patients for ongoing studies [1]. Due to patients moving between different services and clinical areas, ward staff may be unable or sometimes unwilling to meet the additional requirements to retain a research patient, such as increased monitoring, ongoing sample collections, or screening [2].

Wong and colleagues identified three main barriers to participating in oncology clinical trials: (1) lack of appropriate trials for community-based settings, (2) insufficient infrastructure support, and (3) increased physician burden. Amongst the main obstacles that the clinicians have tackled, under-involvement in clinical research has been a major barrier to the future of studies. Additionally, the costs of oncology trials are borne by a combination of third-party reimbursement for the cancer care and institution and research study support for the specific costs of the research trials; this can be considered as another obstacle.

The business model for a clinical research programme is very different from the model for running a successful and profitable medical practice in the real world. Relationships with pharmaceutical sponsors, sometimes quavered, can take years to develop. Starting and maintaining a programme can be expensive and time-consuming for beginners. In addition, another recurring problem of this business model is the decentralisation of clinical trials. Currently, 85% of all clinical trials fail to recruit enough patients, a total of 80% of studies are delayed due to recruitment problems, and dropout rates are high.

A relatively new approach called patient-centric trials has helped to address some of these issues. For instance, the Future of Drug Development study by the Economist Intelligence Unit patient-centric trials took an average of 4 months to recruit 100 participants, instead of the typical 7 months required for all the other types of trials. The lack of awareness and inadequate advert campaign around clinical trials are parts of the problem when it comes to addressing low participation, for instance. Socioeconomic, geographic, and financial factors also come into play for potential participants and must be addressed if clinical researchers are to overcome recruitment problems.

Hard work coupled with increased knowledge is essential elements for making clinical trials more accessible to a more diverse population of patients and volunteers. Bio-psycho-social factors such as finance, education, behaviour, and geography still have a limiting influence on those who could participate. Those in the clinical industry should be willing to face the obstacles that stand in the way of these demographics.

15.4 Maximising the digital landscape

Health systems around the world show great diversity in terms of decisions about the implementation of new health technologies and the expectations of service users. Health management requires difficult choices on a daily basis at all levels of the health system. Currently, there are a multitude of interventions in healthcare, being continually expanded with new drugs, equipment, research, and medical procedures.

COVID-19, for example, has represented a major scientific and public health challenge. The need for knowledge about the mechanisms of transmission, prevention, and therapeutic options continues to grow exponentially. The pressure to find the answers to these questions explains the high demand for clinical trials. If, on the one hand, this crisis has hampered the evolution of different means to complete studies, since patients are afraid to travel to the research centre; on the other hand, the pandemic also has brought agility to the regulatory approval of clinical research.

The term digital health has rapidly expanded to encompass a much broader set of scientific concepts and technologies, including genomics, artificial intelligence, analytics, wearables, mobile apps, and telemedicine. In addition, digital health technologies are being applied much more broadly in medicine to include more accurate diagnoses, effective treatment, clinical decision support, care management, and care delivery.

The rapid advancement and promotion of digital healthcare technologies have produced a unique and iconic landscape characterised by an industry capable of rapidly iterating technology, often at the expense of traditional medical product design and clinical efficacy testing. Prior to the digital and mobile era of healthcare technology, the speed of technology development has been defined by manufacturing, distribution, and regulatory considerations, which inherently require a slower development cycle.

References

[1] Apfeld JC, Deans KJ. Learning health systems and the future of clinical research. J Pediatr Surg 2020;55S:51–3. https://doi.org/10.1016/j.jpedsurg.2019.09.009. Epub 2019 Oct 24 31662193.
[2] O'Gara P, Harrington RA. The future of clinical research and the ACC: empowerment through registries, data, and our members. J Am Coll Cardiol 2014;64 (16):1751–2. https://doi.org/10.1016/j.jacc.2014.09.005. 25323264.

Index

Note: Page numbers followed by *f* indicate figures, *t* indicate tables and *b* indicate boxes.

Printed in the United States
by Baker & Taylor Publisher Services